MaXimized Living

MAKEOVER

Published in Orlando, Florida, by Maximized Living Publishing, Inc.

The stories included in this book are based on real examples of real people, although the names were changed. Any similarity between these stories to living persons whose authorization was not received prior to publication is unintentional.

In view of the complex, individual nature of health and fitness problems, this book, and the ideas, programs, procedures, and suggestions are not intended to replace the advice of trained medical professionals. All matters regarding one's health require medical supervision. A physician should be consulted prior to adopting any program or programs described in this book, or any of the Maximized Living resources. The contents of this book are based upon the opinions of the authors. The author and publisher disclaim any liability arising directly or indirectly from the use of this book.

Only your medical doctor can prescribe drugs, tell you to get off of drugs, or provide medical advice. *That's the practice of medicine.* The role of this book is to make you aware of the hazards of poor lifestyle decisions and alert you to the inherent dangers of medications, while helping you to create optimum function and healing in your body.

Library of Congress Cataloging-in-Publication Data

Lerner, Ben; Loman, Greg; Majors, Charles.
   Maximized Living Makeover
     p. cm.
   ISBN 1-933936-56-8
   1. Health   2. Nutrition   3. Happiness
     I. Ben Lerner. II. Title
Printed in the United States of America

MaXimized Living

MAKEOVER

by

Dr. Ben Lerner | Dr. Greg Loman | Dr. Charles Majors

Special Thanks

To you, the reader, for being willing to make the rest of your life the best of your life by making it a

MaXimized Life!

For additional information on Maximized Living, including video enhancement of this book, exercise illustrations, eating plans, resources, and more, please log on to:

www.MaximizedLivingMakeover.com

Contents

Official Maximized Living Doctors

These doctors are widely regarded for their commitment to excellence in health care and their outstanding contributions to Maximized Living.

Drs. Ben and Sheri Lerner
604 Front Street
Celebration, FL 34747
www.maximizedlivingdrBLerner.com

Drs. Greg and Maryella Loman
2515 Northbrooke Plaza Dr., Ste 102
Naples, FL 34119
www.maximizedlivingdrLoman.com

Dr. Charles Majors
432 N Weber Rd.
Romeoville, IL 60446
www.maximizedlivingdrMajors.com

ALABAMA
Dr. Mike Bucknell
921 Tanner Williams Rd., Ste. 1
Mobile, AL 36608
www.maximizedlivingdrBucknell.com

ARIZONA
Drs. Wes and Jackie Hunter
3303 S Lindsay Rd., Ste. 109
Gilbert, AZ 85297
www.maximizedlivingdrHunter.com

CALIFORNIA
Dr. Lucas Odahlen
24875 Prielipp Rd., #214
Wildomar, CA 92595
www.maximizedlivingdrOdahlen.com

COLORADO
Dr. Joe Arvay
10673 Melody Dr.
Northglenn, CO 80234
www.maximizedlivingdrArvay.com

Dr. Tom Bolan
10890 E Dartmouth Ave., Ste. 6
Aurora, CO 80014
www.maximizedlivingdrBolan.com

Dr. Kristen Kells
6285 Lehman Dr., Bldg. D, Ste. 101
Colorado Springs, CO 80918
www.maximizedlivingdrKells.com

Drs. Joel and Kathy Kinch
316 4th St.
Castle Rock, CO 80104
www.maximizedlivingdrKinch.com

Dr. Chris Pellow
6854 S Dallas Way
Greenwood Village, CO 80112
www.maximizedlivingdrPellow.com

Dr. Paul Price
4 W Dry Creek Cir., #125
Littleton, CO 80120
www.maximizedlivingdrPrice.com

Dr. Eric Shuemake
5657 S Himalaya St., #250
Aurora, CO 80015
www.maximizedlivingdrShuemake.com

Drs. Joseph Singh and Kristin Hoffman
2750 S Wadsworth Blvd., C109
Lakewood, CO 80227
www.maximizedlivingdrSingh.com

FLORIDA
Dr. Gary Bolen
4140 Woodmere Park Blvd., Ste. 2
Venice, FL 34293
www.maximizedlivingdrBolen.com

Dr. Matthew Herba
158 Tuskawilla Rd., Ste. 1308
Winter Springs, FL 32708
www.maximizedlivingdrHerba.com

Dr. Erik Lerner
1405-D Hiawassee Rd.
Orlando, FL 32835
www.maximizedlivingdrELerner.com

Dr. Rich Lerner
11241 E Colonial Dr., Ste. 210
Orlando, FL 32817
www.maximizedlivingdrRLerner.com

Dr. Tony Nalda
4041 13th St.
St. Cloud, FL 34769
www.maximizedlivingdrNalda.com

Dr. Scott Stoltz
2101 S Parsons Ave.
Seffner, FL 33584
www.maximizedlivingdrStoltz.com

Dr. Matthew Symons
1011 N State Rd. 7, Ste. D
Royal Palm Beach, FL 33411
www.maximizedlivingdrSymons.com

Drs. Darrin and Shanelle Tyson
920 W Lumsder
Brandon, FL 33511
www.maximizedlivingdrTyson.com

Dr. Dan Yachter
3577 Lake Emma Rd., Ste. 121
Lake Mary, FL 32746
www.maximizedlivingdrYachter.com

GEORGIA
Dr. Mark Domanski
320 E Montgomery Crossroads, #30
Savannah, GA 31406
www.maximizedlivingdrDomanski.com

Dr. Fred Roberto
5041 Dallas Hwy., Ste. 500
Powder Springs, GA 30127
www.maximizedlivingdrRoberto.com

IDAHO
Dr. Rosie Main
317 Happy Day Blvd., Ste. 170
Caldwell, ID 83607
www.maximizedlivingdrMain.com

ILLINOIS
Dr. Shawn Bladel
2807 N Vermilion St., Ste. 1B
Danville, IL 61832
www.maximizedlivingdrBladel.com

Dr. James Judge
2422 W Main St.
St. Charles, IL 60174
www.maximizedlivingdrJudge.com

Dr. Mark Myers
416 E Roosevelt Rd., Ste. 101
Wheaton, IL 60187
www.maximizedlivingdrMyers.com

Dr. Ashly Ochsner
14400 S John Humprey Dr., Ste. 110
Orland Park, IL 60462
www.maximizedlivingdrOchsner.com

Dr. Nathan Thompson
664 W Veterans Parkway, Ste. A
Yorkville, IL 60560
www.maximizedlivingdrThompson.com

KANSAS
Dr. Georgia Ohlberg
737 S Washington, #4
Wichita, KS 67211
www.maximizedlivingdrOhlberg.com

LOUISIANA
Dr. Jason Maggio
8575 Fern Ave., Ste. 100
Shreveport, LA 71105
www.maximizedlivingdrMaggio.com

MICHIGAN
Drs. Derek and Ryan Bittner
13927 Plumbrook Rd.
Sterling Heights, MI 48312
www.maximizedlivingdrBittner.com

Dr. Mark McCullough
243 North Ave.
Battle Creek, MI 49017
www.maximizedlivingdrMcCullough.com

Dr. Chris Niedzinski
30701 W Ten Mile Rd., Ste. 300
Farmington Hills, MI 48336
www.maximizedlivingdrNiedzinski.com

Dr. C. J. Trupp
15614 Farmington Rd.
Livonia, MI 48154
www.maximizedlivingdrTrupp.com

MINNESOTA
Dr. Brenda Kress
333 Grand Ave., Ste. 102
St. Paul, MN 55102
www.maximizedlivingdrKress.com

Dr. Erik Okeson
16372 Kenrick Ave., Ste. 210
Lakeville, MN 55044
www.maximizedlivingdrOkeson.com

Dr. Jeff Styba
10950 Club West Pkwy., Ste. 110
Blaine, MN 55449
www.maximizedlivingdrStyba.com

Dr. Pete Wurdemann
6368 Elm St., PO Box 94
North Branch, MN 55056
www.maximizedlivingdrWurdemann.com

MISSOURI
Dr. Amanda Campbell
108 SW Blue Pkwy.
Lees Summit, MO 64063
www.maximizedlivingdrCampbell.com

Dr. Jessica Hoffman
355 Mid Rivers Mall Dr., Ste. C
St. Peters, MO 63376
www.maximizedlivingdrHoffman.com

MISSISSIPPI
Dr. Ryan Miller
761 Rice Rd., Apt. 1320
Ridgeland, MS 39157
www.maximizedlivingdrMiller.com

NORTH CAROLINA
Dr. Lonnie Ragwell
10310 Feldfarm Ln., Ste. 100
Charlotte, NC 28210
www.maximizedlivingDrfrancisDrBagwell.com

Dr. Jessica Bohon
13504 Pacific Echo Dr.
Charlotte, NC 28277
www.maximizedlivingdrBohon.com

Dr. Charles Francis
10310 Feldfarm Ln., Ste. 100
Charlotte, NC 28210
www.maximizedlivingDrfrancisDrBagwell.com

Drs. Brent and Daphne Maxwell
10215A Hickorywood Hill Ave.
Huntersville, NC 28078
www.maximizedlivingdrMaxwell.com

Drs. Marc and Joelle Surprenant
7245 Pineville-Matthews Rd., Ste. 300
Charlotte, NC 28226
www.maximizedlivingdrSurprenant.com

NEBRASKA
Dr. Dan Sullivan
1600 Normandy Ct., Ste. 110
Lincoln, NE 68512
www.maximizedlivingdrSullivan.com

NEW YORK
Dr. Eric Ashburn
209 Old Route 9
Fishkill, NY 12524
www.maximizedlivingdrAshburn.com

Dr. Tom Kovacs
48 East 43rd St., 4th Floor
New York, NY 10017
www.maximizedlivingdrKovacs.com

PENNSYLVANIA
Dr. Dan Pompa
145 Lake Dr., Ste. 104
Wexford, PA 15090
www.maximizedlivingdrPompa.com

SOUTH CAROLINA
Dr. Justin James
455 Trolley Rd.
Summerville, SC 29485
www.maximizedlivingdrJames.com

Dr. Dwyer Scott
3705 Renee Dr.
Myrtle Beach, SC 29579
www.maximizedlivingdrScott.com

TENNESSEE
Dr. Alan Arstikaitis
7870 Winchester Rd.
Memphis, TN 38125
www.maximizedlivingdrArstikaitis.com

Dr. Joshua Axe
15123 Old Hickory Blvd.
Nashville, TN 37212
www.maximizedlivingdrAxe.com

Dr. Dionne Kellogg
1746 General George Patton Dr., Ste. 102
Brentwood, TN 37027
www.maximizedlivingdrKellogg.com

Drs. Jason and Jenny Kestner
5964 Temple Rd.
Nashville, TN 37221
www.maximizedlivingdrKestner.com

TEXAS
Dr. John Ensign
11120 Shallow Water Rd.
Austin, TX 78717
www.maximizedlivingdrEnsign.com

Drs. David and Kimberly Erb
10009 N MacArthur Blvd., Ste. 109
Irving, TX 75063
www.maximizedlivingdrErb.com

Dr. Randy Johns
3316 Richmond Rd.
Texarkana, TX 75503
www.maximizedlivingdrJohns.com

Drs. Jimmy and Tiffany Labrecque
7948 Davis Blvd.
N Richland Hills, TX 76180
www.maximizedlivingdrLabrecque.com

Dr. Mick Mahan
16259 FM 529
Houston, TX 77095
www.maximizedlivingdrMahan.com

Dr. Michael McCracken
300 E Round Grove Rd., Apt. 0311
Lewisville, TX 75067
www.maximizedlivingdrMcCracken.com

Dr. Kyle Meers
607 Chandler Branch
Leander, TX 78641
www.maximizedlivingdrMeers.com

Dr. Eric Narrell
4119 Wolflin
Amarillo, TX 79102
www.maximizedlivingdrNarrell.com

Dr. Rob Vasquez
2044 Bedford Rd.
Bedford, TX 76021
www.maximizedlivingdrVasquez.com

Dr. Aaron Wall
3250 Huler St., Apt. 140
Fort Worth, TX 76107
www.maximizedlivingdrWall.com

WASHINGTON
Dr. Troy Dreiling
9418 NE Vancouver Mall Dr., Ste. 101
Vancouver, WA 98662
www.maximizedlivingdrDreiling.com

WISCONSIN
Dr. Emmett Blahnik
7836 Mineral Point Rd.
Madison, WI 53717
www.maximizedlivingdrBlahnik.com

Dr. Jason Lang
4070 W Spencer St.
Appleton, WI 54914
www.maximizedlivingdrLang.com

CANADA
Dr. Joel Bohemier
154 Provencher Blvd.
Winnipeg, MB R2H 0G3
www.maximizedlivingdrBohemier.com

Dr. Colin Elkin
160 Brant Ave.
Brantford, ON N3T 3H7
www.maximizedlivingdrElkin.com

Dr. B. J. Hardick
331 Queens Ave.
London, ON N6B 1X2
www.maximizedlivingdrHardick.com

Dr. Jeff Winchester
52 Bridgeport Rd. E
Waterloo, ON N2J 2J6
www.maximizedlivingdrWinchester.com

Official Maximized Living Mentors

These doctors are trusted providers of the science and principles of Maximized Living.

ALABAMA
Dr. Patty Long
Long Chiropractic
12036 Hwy 231-431 N, Ste. A
Meridianville, AL 35759

Drs. Kyle and Renee Lopez
Lopez Family Chiropractic
401 N Section St.
Fairhope, AL 36532

ARKANSAS
Dr. Eric Bailey
Bailey Health Center
125 Main Street SE, Ste. A
Gravette, AR 72736

Dr. Philip Bland
NWA Chiropractic
2102 W Pleasant Grove Rd., Ste. 2
Rogers, AR 72758

ARIZONA
Dr. Michael Dahl
2622 N Steves Blvd.
Flagstaff, AZ 86004

Dr. David Stender
Living Well Chiropractic
6595 N Oracle Road, #135
Tucson, AZ 85704

Dr. Emil Tompkins
7620 N Heartman Ln., Ste. 124-2
Tucson, AZ 85743

CALIFORNIA
Dr. David Barton
Barton Chiropractic
1251 Monument Blvd., Ste. 140
Concord, CA 94520

Dr. Jeffery Gancas
River City Chiropractic
7508 Sunrise Blvd.
Citrus Heights, CA 95610

Dr. Nicholas Houston
16161 Ventura Blvd., #227
Encino, CA 91436

Dr. Kenneth Moger
River City Chiropractic
7508 Sunrise Blvd.
Citrus Heights, CA 95610

COLORADO
Dr. Zack Alme
The Life House
2770 Dagny Way, Ste. 114
Lafayette, CO 80026

Dr. Jess Baldwin
Saddle Rock Chiropractic Center
5657 S Himalyaya St., #280
Centennial, CO 80015

Dr. Michael Cadwallader
Enjoy Great Health Chiropractic
2030 E County Line Rd., Unit U
Highlands Ranch, CO 80126

Dr. David Lee Coleman
Quick Gym
6040 N Carefree Cir.
Colorado Springs, CO 80922

Dr. Tim Cummins
Infinity Wellness Center
1080 S Sable Blvd.
Aurora, CO 80012

Dr. Dustin Ferrell
Optimal Health Chiropractic
12995 Sheridan Blvd., #101
Broomfield, CO 80020

Dr. Nate Irwin
2531 S Shields St., Ste. 2J
Fort Collins, CO 80526

Dr. Ty Johnson
Chiro Connection
3425 Austin Bluffs Pkwy., #110
Colorado Springs, CO 80918

Dr. Keppen Laszlo
Discover Chiropractic
8410 Wadsworth
Arvada, CO 80003

Dr. John Lloyd
5191 S Yosemite, A
Greenwood Village, CO 80111

Dr. Kevin Noffsinger
New Hope Family Chiropractic
10200 E Gerard Ave., Ste. C-147
Denver, CO 80231

Dr. Nancy Pederson
Pederson Chiropractic
20128 E Dartmouth Dr.
Aurora, CO 80013

Dr. Susie Rivard
Essential Chiropractic
Neurology Center
1814 N Wahsatch Ave.
Colorado Springs, CO 80907

Dr. Ron Salvaggione
Alta Vista Chiropractic
4675 Centennial Blvd.
Colorado Springs, CO 80919

Dr. Christie Sonchar
Chiropractic Solutions
1750 Telstar Dr., Ste. 201
Colorado Springs, CO 80920

Dr. Doug Terry
2960 Diagonal Hwy., #206
Boulder, CO 80301

DELAWARE
Dr. Susan Coe
32 Sarazen Dr.
Middletown, DE 19709

Dr. Brian Mowll
Delaware Chiropractic
6-B Trolley Sq.
Wilmington, DE 19806

FLORIDA
Dr. Joe Accurso III
Abundant Life Wellness Center
9040 SW 152 St.
Miami, FL 33157

Dr. Julio Anta
Anta's Fitness and Self Defense
9956 NW 51 Terr.
Miami, FL 33178

Dr. Tim Bassett
Bassett Family Chiropractic
201 Florida Place SE
Fort Walton Beach, FL 32548

Dr. Frank Berzanskis
Lake Nona Family Chiropractic
10743 Narcoossee Rd., Ste. A12
Orlando, FL 32832

Dr. Peter Camiolo
9141 Carolina Ave.
Bonita Springs, FL 34135

Dr. Tessie Carter
5667 CR 577
Center Hill, FL 33514

Dr. Foster Cullum
Cullum Chiropractic
1427 S 3rd St.
Jacksonville Beach, FL 32250

Dr. Frank Curto
1712 Split Fork Dr.
Oldsmar, FL 34677

Dr. Paul Eakle
Bethel Assembly of God
3023 W Patterson St.
Tampa, FL 33614

Dr. Scott Ewing
Chiropractic Associates
705 W John Sims Pkwy.
Niceville, FL 32578

Dr. Dean Jacks
Chiropractic Associates
705 W John Sims Pkwy.
Niceville, FL 32578

Dr. Timothy Jay
Corrective Care Chiropractic
4517 26th St. W
Bradenton, FL 34207

Dr. Matthew McAlees
Palmer Florida
796 Pheasant Run Ct.
Port Orange, FL 32127

Dr. Thomas Myers
World Class Chiropractic
27732 Cashford Cir., Ste. 101
Wesley Chapel, FL 33543

Dr. Michael Norman
Big Pine Key Chiropractic
207 Key Deer Blvd.
Big Pine Key, FL 33043

Dr. Chad Rechcygl
Palmer Florida
5460 Landis Ave.
Port Orange, FL 32127

Dr. Roger Romano
Romano Family Chiropractic
1575 North Lockwood Ridge Rd.
Sarasota, FL 34237

Dr. Sean Savedoff
Savedoff Family Chiropractic
Center
7110 SW 40th St.
Miami, FL 33155

Dr. Jay Seltzer
Seltzer Family Chiropractic
741 Maitland Ave.
Altamonte Springs, FL 32701

Dr. Mike Shaub
Palmer Florida
PO Box 291391
Port Orange, FL 32129

Dr. Michael Sosa
Westchase Chiropractic
10981 Countryway Blvd.
Tampa, FL 33626

Dr. Patrick St. Germain
St. Germain Chiropractic
877 South Orange Blossom Trail
Apopka, FL 32703

Dr. David Yachter
Champion Chiropractic
10189 Cleary Blvd. Ste. 103
Plantation, FL 33324

GEORGIA
Dr. Michael Huppert
Five Points Chiropractic
920 S. Milledge Ave.
Athens, GA 30605

Dr. Chad Hyatt
Hyatt Family Chiropractic
105 Satellite Blvd., Ste. D
Suwanee, GA 30024

Dr. David Jockers
Life University
805 Huntington Rd., Apt. 3
Marietta, GA 30060

Dr. Chris Lockerman
Lockerman Family Chiropractic
1899 Lake Rd., Ste. 113
Hiram, GA 30141

Dr. Eric Richards
HealthSprout Chiropractic
180 Towne Lake Pkwy.
Woodstock, GA 30188

Dr. Nick Sudano
Sudano Family Chiropractic
4401 Shallowford Rd., #142
Roswell, GA 30075

IOWA
Dr. Bryce Armstrong
New Life Chiropractic
502 N Ankeny Blvd., Ste. 5
Ankeny, IA 50023

Dr. David Diehl
Diehl Chiropractic
700 Main St., Ste. 213
Pella, IA 50219

Dr. Scott Richmond
Elite Spinal Rehab, PC
2753 86th St.
Urbandale, IA 50322

Dr. Jeffery Stickel
Stickel Chiropractic Clinic
2913 Ingersoll Ave.
Des Moines, IA 50312

Dr. Abigail Tebbe
Health From Within
4855 Asbury Rd., Ste. 6
Dubuque, IA 52001

IDAHO
Dr. Doug Brewer
Blue Mountain Chiropractic
280 E. Corporate Dr., Ste. 130
Meridian, ID 83642

Dr. Justin Griffin
2016 S Eagle Rd.
Meridian, ID 83642

ILLINOIS
Dr. Curt Buss
Harmony Chiropractic
584 Randall Rd.
South Elgin, IL 60177

Dr. Bryon Coker
Family Health Chiropractic
1736 Essington Rd., Ste. C
Joliet, IL 60435

Dr. Nathan Conroy
The Chiropractic People
1881 S Randall Rd.
Geneva, IL 60134

Dr. David Foss
Vital Chiropractic
108 Valley Dr., F
Elburn, IL 60119

Dr. Andrew Hajduk
Chiropractic Health Centre
131 E Townline Rd.
Vernon Hills, IL 60061

Dr. Richard Hyde
Complete Chiropractic
416 E Roosevelt Rd., Ste. 108
Wheaton, IL 60187

Dr. Matthew Milonas
Milonas Family Chiropractic
1603 N Aurora Rd., Ste. 111
Naperville, IL 60563

Dr. Paul Stoetzel
Stoetzel's Planet Chiropractic
1192 Walter St., Ste. C
Lemont, IL 60439

Dr. Tim Weselak
Lombard Chiropractic
1127 S. Main St.
Lombard, IL 60148

INDIANA
Dr. Karen Bisesi
Indy Sports Chiropractic
1021 S Rangelkine Rd.
Carmel, IN 46032

Dr. Brean Symmonds
Indy Sports and Family
Chiropractic
75 Executive Dr., Ste. J
Carmel, IN 46032

KANSAS
Dr. Michael Cortner
Cortner Chiropractic Clinic
1109 Waters St.
Manhattan, KS 66503

KENTUCKY
Dr. Michael Redman
Chiropractic Family Wellness
7276 Burlington Pike
Florence, KY 41042

MASSACHUSETTS
Dr. Gerry Cassista
Cassista Chiropractic Office
1350 Lakeview Ave.
Dracut, MA 01826

Dr. Allison Glass
Deerfield Family Chiropractic
267 Amherst Rd., Ste. 1
Sunderland, MA 01375

MICHIGAN
Dr. Ronson Dykstra
Dykstra Chiropractic
3083 Washington Ave. SW, Ste. D
Grandville, MI 49418

Dr. Mary Frye
1st Chiropractic Life Center
12445 E 12 Mile Rd.
Warren, MI 48093

Dr. Ed McCuiston
Touch of Life
46755 Hayes Rd.
Shelby Township, MI 48315

Dr. John McLean
McLean Family Chiropractic
1208 N 3rd Street
Marquette, MI 49855

Dr. Gabriel O'Brien
O'Brien Family Chiropractic Center
1519 E River Rd., Ste. B
Muskegon, MI 49445

Dr. Chris O'Dell
O'Dell Chiropractic Center
5454 Carroll Lake Rd.
Commerce Twp, MI 48382

Dr. J. R. VanderWall
Dykstra Chiropractic
3083 Washington Ave. SW, Ste. D
Grandville, MI 49418

Dr. Rhonda VanderWall
Dykstra Chiropractic
3083 Washington Ave. SW, Ste. D
Grandville, MI 49418

Dr. Michael Wegmann
Discover Chiropratic
2000 Harbor Petoskey Rd.
Petoskey, MI 49770

MINNESOTA
Dr. Brian Arvold
Arvold Chiropractic
5685 Geneva Ave. N
Oakdale, MN 55128

Dr. Joel Fugleberg
HealthQuest Chiropractic and
Wellness Center
7945 Stone Creek Dr., Ste. 120
Chanhassen, MN 55317

Dr. Jason Gerard
Lakewoods Chiropractic
255 Highway 97, Ste. 2A
Forest Lake, MN 55025

Dr. Phil Gilman
Lifespring Chiropractic
4640 Slater Rd., Ste. 100
St. Paul, MN 55122

Dr. Nick Krause
Chiropractic First Wellness Center
2518 Superior Dr. NW, Ste. 101B
Rochester, MN 55901

Dr. Bradley Kuehl
Corrective Care Chiropractic
922 125th Ln. NE
Blaine, MN 55434

Dr. ShaRhae Angela Matousek
Real Health Chiropractic Clinic
8901 Aztec Dr.
Eden Prairie, MN 55347

Official Maximized Living Mentors

[Continued]

Dr. Aaron Morland
Valeo Health and Wellness
470 W 78th St., Ste. 120
Chanhassen, MN 55317

Dr. Tony Parks
Chiropractic First Wellness Center
2518 Superior Dr. NW, Ste. 101B
Rochester, MN 55901

Dr. Warren Zook
Adjust to Health Chiropractic
3 W Highway 55, #5A
Buffalo, MN 55313

MISSOURI
Dr. Chris Long
Adjust 4 Life
101 Doc Henry
Greenwood, MO 64034

MONTANA
Dr. Spence Jahner
We Care Chiropractic
804 N 19th Ave.
Bozeman, MT 59718

NORTH CAROLINA
Dr. Joy McClenny
Family Chiropractic Plus
4870-1 Long Beach Rd.
Southport, NC 28461

Dr. Terri Wells
Family First Chiropractic
PO Box 1945
Shallotte, NC 28459

NEBRASKA
Dr. Linn Erickson
5757 S 34th St., #300
Lincoln, NE 68516

NEW JERSEY
Dr. Brad Butler
Chiropractic Works
306 Ramapo Valley Rd.
Oakland, NJ 07436

Dr. Douglas Kaner
Kaner Family Chiropractic
23-08 Maple Ave.
Fairlawn, NJ 07410

Dr. Fred Rossi
Rossi Family Chiropractic
1072 Valley Rd.
Stirling, NJ 07980

Dr. Robert White
True Health Chiropractic
442 Morris Ave.
Springfield, NJ 07081

NEW YORK
Dr. Brian Bartholomew
PO Box 11
Lansing, NY 14882

Dr. Daniel Golaszewski
New York Chiropractic College
129 Juniper Rd.
Kings Park, NY 11754

LoriRene Koehn
#8 Warren St.
Albany, NY 12203

OHIO
Dr. Jay Villella
Lane Avenue Chiropractic
1301 W Lane Ave.
Columbus, OH 43221

OKLAHOMA
Dr. Lance Bailey
Bailey Chiropractic
5840 S Memorial, Ste. 307
Tulsa, OK 74145

Dr. David Dick
Body by God Chiropractic
Sanctuary
1157 S Aspen Ave.
Broken Arrow, OK 74012

Dr. Matt Ford
4301 NW 63rd, Ste. 102
Oklahoma City, OK 73116

Dr. Ryan Hanson
Hanson Chiropractic Center
1717 South Blvd., Ste. B
Edmond, OK 73013

PENNSYLVANIA
Dr. Steve Mustin
Mustin Chiropractic
69 N Wren Drive
Pittsburgh, PA 15243

Dr. Richard Schaffnit
11730 E Main Rd.
North East, PA 16428

SOUTH CAROLINA
Dr. Rachelle Larsen
Coastal Chiropractic Center
5401 Netherby Ln., Ste. 201
North Charleston, SC 29420

Dr. Heather Wyant
Atlantic Coast Chiropractic
613 Old Trolley Rd., Ste. B
Summerville, SC 29485

Dr. Sonya Young
Elite Chiropractic
3 Southridge Ln.
Wrightsville Beach, SC 28480

TENNESSEE
Dr. Seven Aungst
Back to Wellness Chiropractic
2149 W Emory Rd.
Powell, TN 37849

Dr. Zsolt Muller
Health 4 Life Chiropractic
2805 D Old Fort Pkwy.
Murfreesboro, TN 37128

Dr. David Shreve
Bearden Chiropractic Clinic
6725 Papermill Rd.
Knoxville, TN 37919

Dr. Chad Upchurch
Life Source Chiropractic
491 Henslee Dr.
Dickson, TN 37055

TEXAS
Dr. Charles Barnwell
Chiropractic Plus
4500-D N Highway 6
Houston, TX 77084

Dr. Laura Biles
Biles Family Chiropractic
100 Executive Ct., Ste. 1
Waxahachie, TX 75165

Dr. Josh Bonine
Parker College
1315 Riverchase Dr., #815
Coppell, TX 75019

Dr. Bo Brantley
Brantley Chiropractic of
McKinney
1203 W University Dr.
McKinney, TX 75069

Dr. Brian Hooten
Hooten Family Chiropractic
16970 Dallas Pkwy., # 201
Dallas, TX 75248

Dr. William Hopson
Hopson Chiropractic
1404 Rice Rd., Ste. 400
Tyler, TX 75703

Dr. Teresa Jones
Whole Health Chiropractic
3930 Naaman School Rd., Ste. B
Garland, TX 75040

Dr. Matthew Karcher
Discover Complete Wellness
5646 Milon St., Ste. 537
Dallas, TX 75206

Dr. Brian Nimphius
Infinity Chiropractic
3001 N Main St., #250
Euless, TX 76039

Dr. Ben Spitzenberger
Irving, TX 75063

Dr. Jimmy Vanderburg
Labrecque Family Chiropractic
8304 Oak Ct.
North Richland Hills, TX 76180

UTAH
Dr. Tiffani Fries
Genesis Chiropractic
715 E 3900 So., Ste. 201
Salt Lake City, UT 84107

WASHINGTON
Dr. Tye Bratvold
Millenium Chiropractic
702 South Hill Park Dr., Ste. 101
Puyallup, WA 98373

Dr. Cyrus Dohrmann
Dohrmann Family Chiropractic
2321 Simpson Ave.
Aberdeen, WA 98520

Dr. John Wood
Live Well Chiropractic
12950 SE Kent Kangley Rd.
Kent, WA 98030

Dr. Tim Yoder
Back to Health Chiropractic
16111 SE McGillvray Blvd.
Vancouver, WA 98683

WISCONSIN
Dr. Krista Bohling
901 Aubin St., Lot 54
Peshtigo, WI 54157

Dr. Donald Hundt
Hundt Chiropractic
19035 W Capitol Dr.
Brookfield, WI 53045

Dr. Andrew Treutelaar
Waukesha Chiropractic and Rehab
628 W Moreland Blvd.
Waukesha, WI 53188

CANADA
Dr. Richard Gray
36-550 University Dr. W
Lethbridge, AB T1J 4T3

Dr. Kale Matovich
3527 18th St. SW
Calgary, AB T2T 4T9

Dr. Michael Banman
Rhino Chiropractic
1940 Kane Rd., Ste. 122
Kelowna, BC V1V 2J9

Dr. Brian Bittle
Lifestyle Chiropractic
210-1640 Leckie Rd.
Kelowna, BC V1X 7C6

Dr. Jo'anne Blackman
Mike's Boot Camp
PO Box 20263
Kelowna, BC V1Y 9H2

Dr. Chris Stratis
Stratis Fitness Solutions
PO Box 20263
Kelowna, BC V1Y 9H2

Dr. Mike Stratis
Mike's Boot Camp
PO Box 20263
Kelowna, BC V1Y 9H2

Dr. Jason Wiebe
Summit Chiropractic Studio
Landmark Tower III
#530-1632 Dickson Ave.
Kelowna, BC V1Y 7T2

Dr. Christian Chatzoglou
Chiropractic Life Centre
1431 Corydon Ave.
Winnipeg, MB R3N 0J2

Dr. Tyler Jones
Alpha Chiropractic
1460 Belcher St.
Port Williams, NS B0P 1T0

Dr. Sean Batte
Forest City Family Chiropractic
440 Boler Rd., Ste. 101
London, ON N6K 4L2

Dr. Yurij Chewpa
Warrior Coaching
1195-A Hunt Club Rd.
Ottawa, ON K1V 8S4

Dr. David Covey
2016 Tenth Line, Unit 7
Orleans, ON K4A 4X4

Dr. Mark Del Cantero
201 Wilson St. E, Ste. 111
Ancaster, ON L9G 2B8

Dr. Graham Jenkins
York River Chiropractic Center
194 Hastings St. N, PO Box 419
Bancroft, ON K0L 1C0

Dr. Jim Kaminski
Fergus Family Chiropractic
198 St. David St. N
Fergus, ON N1M 2J6

Dr. Ian McIntosh
1195-A Hunt Club Rd.
Ottawa, ON K1V 8S4

Dr. Brian Nantais
Nantais Family Chiropractic
1614 Lesperance, Unit #3
Tecumseh, ON N8N 1Y3

Dr. Richard Penney
1581 Greenbank Rd.
Ottawa, ON K2J 4Y6

Dr. Ed Quirk
1195-A Hunt Club Rd.
Ottawa, ON K1V 8S4

Dr. Jonathan Saunders
Chiropractic on Eagle
407 Eagle St.
Newmarket, ON L3Y 1K5

Dr. Denise Tomlin
3058 Pettigrew Cres.
Mississauga, ON L5L 4W9

CONTRIBUTING AUTHORS

Special thanks to the following health authorities who provided materials for this book.

Barbara Loe Fisher
Cofounder and president, National Vaccine Information Center
www.nvic.org
www.909shot.com

Dr. Joel Kinch
316 4th St.
Castle Rock, CO 80104
www.maximizedlivingdrKinch.com

Dr. Erik Lerner
1405-D Hiawassee Rd.
Orlando, FL 32835
www.maximizedlivingdrELerner.com

Dr. Tony Nalda
4041 13th St.
Saint Cloud, FL 34769
www.maximizedlivingdrNalda.com

Gwen Olsen
Author of *Confessions of an Rx Drug Pusher*
www.gwenolsen.com

Dr. Ashly Ochsner
14400 S John Humphrey Dr., Ste. 110
Orland Park, IL 60462
www.maximizedlivingdrOchsner.com

Dr. Dan Pompa, DC and Warren P. Phillips, MS.
145 Lake Dr., Ste 104
Wexford, PA 15090
www.maximizedlivingdrPompa.com

Dr. Dan Yachter
3577 Lake Emma Rd., Ste. 121
Lake Mary, FL 32746
www.maximizedlivingdrYachter.com

Introduction
by Dr. Ben Lerner

We have one mission: to save millions of lives through Maximized Living.

Where's Superman? Where's Spiderman? Where's Wonder Woman? Where's Batman? Don't you feel like the world could use a superhero—or two—right about now? At this point, I'd settle for Mighty Mouse or Wonder Dog. Even Scooby Doo and Shaggy would be nice. Somebody to save us...

It's hard to find a happy person right now. With approximately forty million Americans suffering from depression and antidepressants being the leading drugs sold today, plus another forty million people who can't sleep, clearly despair has permeated the masses.

Add to that the long list of other extremely common maladies that plague us like Alzheimer's, diabetes, learning disorders, obesity, chronic fatigue syndrome, allergies, fibromyalgia, high blood pressure, high cholesterol, severe pain, heart disease, cancer, etc., etc., etc., and you wonder if anyone at all is well.

Aquaman, Tarzan, Flash... Someone with super powers is going to have to turn this around. Obviously, modern medicine, modern foods, and modern living aren't going to help. In fact, those are the things we need the most protection from so we don't keep acquiring modern disease.

After writing two *New York Times* best-selling books, being a doctor for two U.S. Olympic teams and the NBA's Orlando Magic, plus speaking all over the world, I've had great chance to see what must change if millions of lives are to be saved.

Along with my coauthors, Dr. Greg Loman (also a *New York Times* best-selling author) and Dr. Charles Majors (one of the most successful doctors of any kind in the world today), we have taken care of literally millions of families. They are families who now have the opportunity to experience maximized living.

Unfortunately, none of us can fly, lift cars, or see through walls like superheroes. But, if you saw how well our families and our patients do vs. the rest of the world's population today, you might think that we could.

We're not heroes—not by a long shot. Neither are the hundreds of other doctors who are out there practicing according to the Maximized Living model. The model, however, does work heroically. It saves lives. Additionally, the work we do that you'll read about in this book, doesn't require leaping over tall buildings in a single bound. It simply requires knowing how you're supposed to live and organize your life vs. the way nearly everyone else is doing it.

You don't want to do what everyone else is doing. In fact, you should do the opposite (see "The Law of Reversal"). Clearly, your mind, your body, and your life will all do far better if you don't conform to the ways of this world and the culture at large.

Just like we've done for millions of people all over the world, we're going to show you how to make over your life, to go from modern living to maximized living.

This is not just another diet-and-exercise book that tells you to work harder at being healthy. In fact, this book proves that living the maximized life is actually *less* work and burden than the unhealthy alternative. And while the vast majority of Americans have chosen that alternative (which is eventually lethal), you can discover a new way of thinking and living that will help you beat the odds and enjoy a long, quality life.

I'm not suggesting it will be easy to change old habits and incorrect thinking. But once you break free of those old patterns and feel the momentum and freedom of the maximized life—you will never want to turn back.

No matter what your age is now, the time to make a change is today. If you are ready for that transformation, this book will be your companion and your guide along the way.

The final section is a step-by-step, day-by-day course of reasonable action and challenges to get you far down the lesser-traveled path of maximized living. Whether you are a beginner or advanced, we will challenge you to embrace a life that is more aligned for health and energy—and even gain stronger relationships and peace of mind.

So if you've ever wondered, "What else is there?" or thought, "There has to be more," Maximized Living is it—and there definitely is!

TAKE A STEP FORWARD!

The book that you hold in your hands is actually a powerful system to guide you through a transforming process that will affect every area of your life. Each chapter ends with practical steps that break the huge strides forward into a series of small, sequenced actions that anyone can do.

This book is:

1. A transformation manual.

2. Your key to a living community at www.MaximizedLivingMakeover.com which is full of special videos, tests, calculators, articles, testimonies, and opportunities for you to share your thoughts—and read the thoughts of others.

3. Instruction from a skilled Maximized Living expert. You may have purchased this book in conjunction with a class being taught by one. If not, you don't want to miss the chance for personal, personalized instruction from a Maximized Living expert. Visit the website to find the one nearest you.

Take a moment now to familiarize yourself with the book. As you can see, it is a unique combination of tools designed to lead you into Maximized Living step by step.

1. The first element is dynamic instruction designed to help you understand the Five Essentials of Maximized Living, and how they all work together to create outrageous health and incredible happiness. Along the way you'll find images that point you to resources on the website that will let you discover more about Maximized Living.

2. The second element consists of three 30-day Challenges, carefully designed for people at the basic, intermediate, and elite levels. Be sure to check with your physician before beginning any of the challenges. Be realistic about where you are. If you're at the basic level, start at the basic level—not the intermediate level. Remember, Maximized Living is walked out one day at a time—for a lifetime. You have plenty of time to advance to the next level.

3. The third element is a meal plan with both basic and advanced levels. Each meal plan gives you over a month of ideas—and not just for the major meals — it also includes suggestions for snacks! You will find even more ideas on the website. There you will find actual recipes and resources to purchase the ingredients.

Take a moment now to familiarize yourself with the website at
www.MaximizedLivingMakeover.com.

You will find it to be the fastest, most efficient way to find resources and encouragement for your journey to a maximized life. Refer to it often. You will find the content informative, the diagnostics illuminating, and the testimonies inspiring!

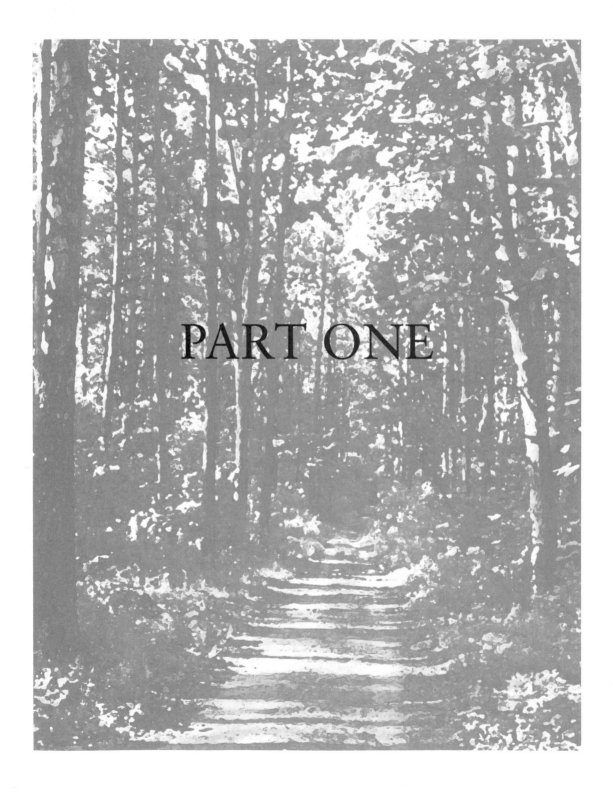

PART ONE

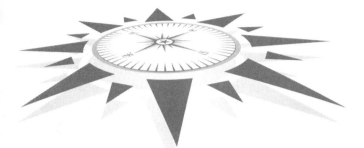

A Journey into Truth, Health, and Freedom

Will you still be alive at sixty? If so, will you just be breathing or will you be living life to the fullest?

If you're living, will you be a walking, talking pharmacy and pincushion, spending your retirement on prescription pills, shots, and hip-replacement surgery? Or will you be enjoying life's rewards like traveling the world and spoiling your grandkids?

When it comes to the thought that you won't make it in good health to the age of sixty, you probably think like many of us: "It's not going to be me!" But in reality, it's almost everyone. It probably is going to be you.

You might also be saying, "What do I care? I'm only twenty-one or thirty-eight. What does that have to do with me?" Well, it has plenty to do with you—right now! Listen to the voices from the grave whispering, "Take care of your youth, or you will lose it and suffer at sixty like we did—if you even make it to sixty!"

If you are like most of your friends, family, and neighbors, you expect to be alive and well at sixty. But the reality is that only an estimated one out of a thousand Americans will celebrate their sixtieth birthday in excellent health, free of medications and feeling good. If you are in America, living by the Western model, your chance of even surviving past sixty is among the worst in the world.[1]

Perhaps you expect that both you *and* your spouse will be healthy and feeling great at sixty. And while that is entirely possible, you will be in the tiny minority if you do. With only one in a thousand individuals doing well at sixty, you can estimate that only one in ten thousand couples will do so.

Every couple's dream is to spend their latter years walking hand in hand down the beach, taking the grandkids to Disney World, enjoying life, participating in hobbies, and still fulfilling a purpose. The fact of the matter is, however, it's probably not going to happen. Look at where you are now. Are you leading the kind of life and experiencing the level of good health that will give you a wonderful future? The decisions you're making today determine your chance for well-being at age sixty and beyond.

Disease occurs now. It just kills you later. What you do today, how your body is functioning currently, what drugs you're on at present, and how well you take care of yourself now will determine your future. Most people live today like there will be no tomorrow. And truly, for many Americans, there won't be.

You might be stunned, perplexed, or even depressed by these numbers, especially in the wealthy United States, where access to clinics, hospitals, medicines, and doctors is better than almost any other country on the planet. But is the United States the healthiest country on the planet? Absolutely not! In fact, it's the least. The United States places last in the world in health care, timely medical care, and in the amount of deaths that could be prevented by a health-care system.[2]

⚡Note: The Western lifestyle and the U.S. health-care model have been making their way overseas to other countries. In other words, fast food and fast relief are quickly reaching other parts of the world now. As you can guess, these other countries are quickly catching "down" to us.

Conventional wisdom just doesn't add up. The U.S. medical model is what everyone is doing, yet very, very few people are actually well. Our advice to you: don't do what everyone is doing! Do not simply follow the tide and get sucked into the majority, who throughout history has *always* been wrong. Even when a billion people believe in a really bad idea, it's still a really bad idea. And the way people in the U.S. take care of themselves, the medical model of the Western World, is a really bad idea.

Mark Twain once said, "When you find yourself on the side of the majority, it's time to pause and reflect." So ask yourself now, do you want your marriage, finances, emotions, your fitness, and health to be like everyone else's? Are the people who influence you and the ones you are getting your advice from, experiencing great lives, great health, riches, and awesome relationships? If they're not, STOP LISTENING TO THEM!

You don't want financial advice from a bankrupt financial broker; you don't want marriage advice from someone who's been divorced three times; and you don't want health advice from a doctor who's not healthy, who is overweight, and who studied drugs as the only medical answer.

You may not think you're living in the Western medical model, but you are. And so are your kids, your parents, your aunt, your neighbor, your pastor, and almost everyone around you.

So what do you do about it? We're glad you asked, and we're glad you picked up this book. Because a different model is shared in Maximized Living—a better, right way of living that will truly afford you incredible physical health, mental strength, and marital happiness with far fewer drugs and medical treatments. It's a way of living that will give you true quality of life and purpose for a long, long, long time. Tens of thousands are living this way. And you can too.

Perhaps you consider yourself a hopeless case. We often have patients who think they are genetically doomed for a certain disease or that their health has deteriorated too far to recover, but the facts prove them completely wrong. The International Agency for Research on Cancer and the World Health Organization have concluded that 80 percent of all cancers are attributed to lifestyle *not* genetics. And this is a conservative number. Other studies reveal that as little as two percent of all diseases and conditions have anything to do with genetics or so-called "bad luck." In other words, about 98 percent of all body types, conditions, and disease are due, at least in part, to lifestyle.

Other studies have shown that many people who live to one hundred years old have genes that are supposedly high risk for disease and early death. Yet, they beat the odds. This is great news, because it shows that almost everybody can do something to stay healthy.

Maximized Living Makeover takes you far beyond just gaining a head full of new information. The final section is a step-by-step, day-by-day challenge to get you far down the lesser-traveled path of true maximized living. Whether you are a beginner or advanced, we will challenge you to embrace a life that is better aligned for health and energy—as well as stronger relationships and peace of mind. If you make healthy changes to your lifestyle and embrace the maximized living challenges, you'll be enjoying life for many, many years to come—and you won't end up a walking pharmacy.

TAKE A STEP FORWARD!

Have you ever seen the first Rocky movie? The poster for that movie said, "His whole life was a 1 in a 1,000,000 shot." When it comes to experiencing incredible health and outrageous happiness, which we call Maximized Living, it is uphill all the way, just like Rocky. You are immersed in a culture that produces depression, anxiety, and disease. But, you have already taken the crucial first step by starting your Maximized Living Makeover. As you will learn, Maximized Living is a journey—you won't get there all at once. Incremental change, over time, leads to revolutionary results!

1. To arrive at any destination, you first need to have a good idea of exactly where you are. So be sure to visit www.MaximizedLivingMakeover.com and take the test that will reveal both your real age and your projected life expectancy given where you are right now.

2. Take a moment to reflect on the voices that are speaking into your life. Are people who are in debt giving you financial advice? Are people who are unhappy telling you how to defeat depression and anxiety? Are people who are taking a fist full of prescription drugs telling you how to be healthy? It is vital to start listening to voices that are actually experiencing the outcomes you desire!

One of the best ways to get consistent, comprehensive input on Maximized Living is to make a habit of visiting the website, and even join the online community. There you'll find support for the journey, a sympathetic ear, and real-time information about what's working for others who are on the same path as you.

3. Remember that genetics are not a death sentence. For instance, the fact that a person's father and mother have diabetes might be more about common diet and exercise choices than DNA. Genetics are only a small part of your overall health equation. Be sure to check out the video on epigenetics on the website to learn more.

4. Reflect on your circle of life—the people who depend on you, the people who would be instantly and negatively affected if you were no longer here. The website has a special tool that will help you identify your circle. Remember, your health isn't just about you!

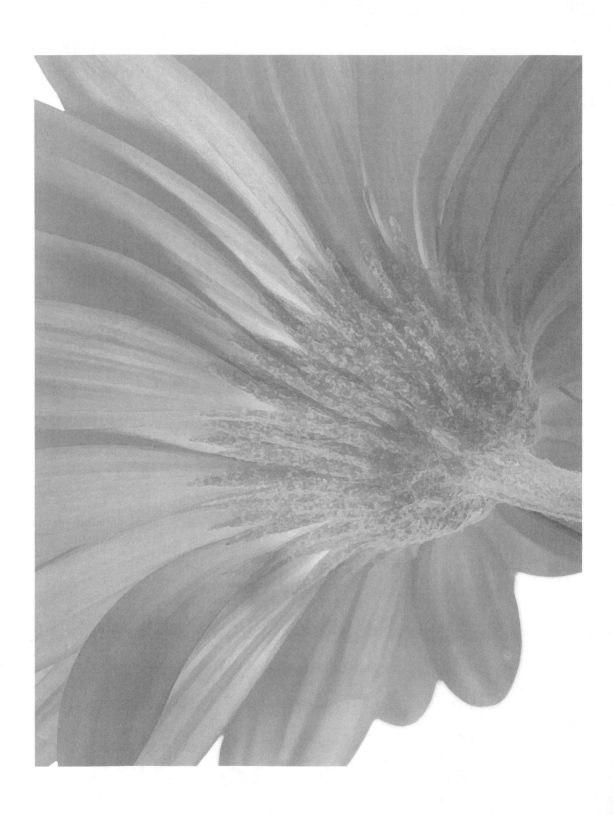

1

Your Body—On Health

While you and most of the people around you have probably been placing your bets on medicine and other artificial schemes to keep you healthy, it's a *bad bet*. You may have very little understanding or appreciation for the healing nature and ability of your own body, so we want to shed some light on the matter for you.

Your body is an amazing, self-healing machine. Ponder for a moment the wonder and majesty of your human body. You are made up of fifty to one hundred trillion cells. You create more than one hundred billion new cells every day of your life. You get new lungs in sixty days, new skin in fourteen days and a new heart in ninety days. You have an arsenal of white blood cells that identify and kill the harmful invaders. Your red blood cells are amazing little vehicles that deliver oxygen to every nook and cranny of your body. Other cells carry electrical impulses that deliver important information to your brain. I could continue, but the point is clear: You are a walking, talking, self-healing wonder. What does this mean for you?

Before we go further, it's important to clarify the definition of true health. Almost everybody would say that if they feel good, then they are healthy. That is a dangerous assumption. People with cancer or blocked arteries or heart disease can feel good. The symptoms

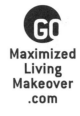

> Your body is an amazing, self-healing machine. You are a walking, talking, self-healing wonder.

MaximizedLivingMakeover.com

TOXICITY TIPS

Kitchen: what to use and what to avoid.

MaximizedLivingMakeover.com

TOXICITY TIPS

Cleaning supplies and common household goods to avoid and best ones to use.

> The symptoms of bad health—not feeling good—will often surface long after the disease begins.

of bad health—not feeling good—will often surface long after the disease begins.

Every common, deadly disease has few or no symptoms in its early stages. Heart disease, cancer, Alzheimer's, arthritis, diabetes, severe pain syndromes, Multiple Sclerosis, and so on do not warn you that they are on their way. With heart disease, for example, the first sign that you have a problem is often that you are dead, which is a little late to start looking into it.

A symptom is the result of cells not functioning properly or not receiving what they have needed for a long time. So utilizing symptoms alone to determine if you're well or not is like jumping off of a high-rise building. As you pass each floor on the way down, you can wave to the people inside and say, "I'm fine," "I'm doing great," "I'm feeling no pain." The symptoms won't show up until you get to the lobby.

Even the best medical tests and regular checkups cannot do much more than detect a disease after it has existed for a while. Medical tests can't prevent any disease; they can only find it after it's there. Early detection is better then late. Unfortunately, at best, it finds sickness early. At worst, it discovers it after—for all intents and purposes—you're already dead.

Finally, the Real Definition of Health

The real definition of health is when all cells of the body are functioning and healing at 100 percent. All disease and even death are caused by groups of your cells not functioning or healing properly.

The fact of the matter is, if your cells are healthy, then so are you. If your cells are weak, sick, not regenerating properly, or dying off too fast, then you are also weak, sick, degenerating, and dying off too fast.

Degenerators Anonymous

Five out of six Americans will die from a degenerative disease. Six out of six will suffer from at least one.

Look around you. Unless the people you know are actively practicing the Essentials of Maximized Living, they're degenerating. It's best to admit it to yourself: "My name is _____, and I'm degenerating."

The unfortunate part of degenerating is that the vast majority of the time it's the fault of the person who is degenerating. It's the way they're living and functioning. That's why many key physicians in the world call degenerative diseases "diseases for dummies."

This is not to insult someone's intelligence; it's simply to point out that degenerative disease is usually the fault of the person who's suffering from it.

If this is you, you know it's true. On some level, you know you're not getting away with certain destructive components in your life. Subconsciously, you know that one day you're going to find yourself on a surgeon's table being given the dreaded cancer diagnosis or in the middle of a heart attack saying, "I knew it!"

Once you admit you're a degenerator, you're ready to make the change.

What Does It Take to Get Healthy?

In order for you to have real health, it's a physical law that the trillions of cells in your body need five elements to function and heal normally, thus, preventing or best healing from disease.

These five essential elements are:
1. Detoxification
2. Nerve Impulse

MaximizedLivingMakeover.com

THE MEDICINE CABINET

The common household 's first line of defense. Read Dr. Ben's report on how we grow up with the medicine cabinet. When we have a headache, a cold, or indigestion, this is usually where we go first. Sometimes the leftovers of old prescriptions become part of the family pharmacy, but there's a better way. For example, since the cause of headaches isn't an aspirin deficiency, wouldn't it be better to find out what's causing the headaches and fix that? In fact, wouldn't it be better to not get headaches in the first place? You won't find the answer in your medicine cabinet. You'll find it here!

> With heart disease, the first sign that you have a problem is often that you are dead.

MEDICINE CABINET DISASTERS

If kids are sneaking your Ritalin, selling your Oxycotin, and getting to sleep with your Xanax, what kind of a disaster is brewing in your medicine cabinet? Read Dr. Charles Majors' report.

BMI CALCULATOR

Look yourself up on the BMI calculator.

BODY TYPE

Check out your body type and locate your body fat. See what this means for your health and what to do about it.

> Medical tests can't prevent any disease; they can only find it after it's there.

3. Nutrients and Water
4. Oxygen and lean muscle
5. Mental/emotional function

What happens if you interfere with these five essential elements?

Toxicity: We all know that you die or get really sick from being poisoned. This includes exposure to chemicals and carcinogens found in medications, vaccines, foods, unhealthy environments, and household cleaning products.

Interference with the central nervous system (CNS): The central nervous system is your brain, spinal cord, and the nerves that run throughout your body. This system is the central computer and master control system of the entire body. If there is disturbance or interference with CNS function, everything breaks down. Emotional stress is one factor that affects, or interferes with, your CNS function. Also, misalignment of the spinal column directly affects and even damages long-term nervous system function.

Nutrient deficiency: As a result of a diet void of necessary nutrients or an inability to absorb nutrients, your body is missing the building blocks it needs to grow new tissue and to heal. It's lacking key chemicals needed for normal physiology.

Oxygen insufficiency: Movement creates the necessary intake of oxygen. Your movement is what transports the oxygen-rich blood through your body, and you become more efficient at the circulation, absorption, and storage of this oxygen. When this happens, your cells have the oxygen they need to survive and live in health. With a sedentary lifestyle, you're literally choking yourself to death.

Fat-to-muscle ratio imbalance: How much fat you have in comparison to lean muscle will be a determining factor in organ function and the development of many common diseases and disorders. By using weight, height, frame, body fat, and muscle analysis, you can determine much about your health and mortality rate.

Mental/emotional stress: Increase in stress hormones creates everything from obesity, high blood pressure, high cholesterol, decreased libido, and aging. Peace is a vital health and longevity necessity in addition to making sure you're not miserable.

It's a Physical Law

> You can't experience health or happiness if you interfere with these five elements no matter what anyone tells you or gives you to swallow!
>
> You can and you will exhibit better health and happiness if you remove interference to these five elements.

The Law of Reversal and the Medical Model

There is an old law called "the law of reversal," which states, "If you want health, wealth, and prosperity, you need to do the exact opposite of what everyone else is doing." (This is also known as the "George Costanza Law." When the character George on the television show *Seinfeld* decided to do everything opposite of usual, his life actually started to get better! He got a job, got a date, and so on.) That adage is absolutely correct when it comes to the way people think and act in regards to their health.

Either by default or by choice, about 99 percent of America's population has embraced what we call the "medical model." The model is based on a set of wrong beliefs and assumptions about our bodies, a misplaced faith in medical technology and drugs, and a blind compliance with whatever our doctor tells us to do.

The truth is stark and clear: The medical model is killing us.

You may think that heart disease, which kills 800,000 people a year, is the greatest killer in America or cancer, which kills 700,000 people a year, but in reality, the number-one cause of death in the United States, killing more than one million people a year, is iatrogenic disease, which simply means *physician-related* disease.

MaximizedLivingMakeover.com

PREMATURE DEATH

In many instances, medicine itself has brought premature death. Read the latest statistics compiled by Dr. Ben Lerner.

The definition of health is when all cells of the body are functioning and healing at 100 percent.
As a result of a diet void of necessary nutrients or an inability to absorb nutrients, your body is missing the building blocks it needs to grow new tissue and to heal.

THE MEDICAL TREADMILL

Medicine gives ailments Latin names. Much of diagnosis is naming instead of treating. Then medicine prescribes a drug to treat a symptom. Learn how to get off the medical tredmill!

THE MEDICAL MARKETING SYNDROME

A special report on restless leg syndrome.

> With a sedentary lifestyle, you literally choke yourself to death.

This includes all of the deaths from some action or drug that is prescribed by a doctor, from going to a hospital, or from surgeries gone bad.

Many doctors know this is true, and even they are fearful of iatrogenic disease. *Time* magazine recently asked a sampling of doctors, surgeons, and pediatricians what scares them the most about being doctors. Their unanimous response: being the patient![3] They were saying, "I would hate to be you and have to go to a doctor!"

These doctors know that doctors can only do two things for you: (1) They can give you drugs (and if that doesn't work, they can give you more drugs). (2) They can do surgery (and if that doesn't work, sometimes more surgery). Today, more and more doctors are admitting that neither drugs nor surgery are the keys to healing.

The title of a recent article in *Business Week* really says it all: "Medical Guesswork: From heart surgery to prostate care, the health industry knows little about which common treatments really work." What does medicine substitute for what works? "Doctors decided whether or not to put a patient in intensive care or use a combination of drugs based on their best judgment and on rules and traditions handed down over the years, as opposed to real scientific proof. These rules and judgments weren't necessarily right."[4]

The traditional drugs that we take—aspirin, blood pressure pills, heart pills, cholesterol pills—are essentially small doses of toxins, administered to bring relief of symptoms. Think about it: what would happen if you swallowed an entire bottle of aspirin or blood pressure pills? You would die, because the chemicals are poisonous. So, if a lot of medication kills you quickly, could it be that small doses over long periods kill you slowly—or at the very least, are not good for you?

By now you may be asking an important question: "Are you telling me to stop going to the doctor and stop taking all my pills?"

We can answer that question by using the analogy of war. Any good military commander knows that using guns and air raids can help win a battle—if the assault is swift and targeted only on the enemy. Similarly, a brief regimen of pills or a surgery may help to win a battle in your body. But here's the problem: pills are often taken indefinitely not for a short period of time, and when people take pills, they are not always "attacking the enemy" as they may suppose. In reality, they are relieving the symptom (the pain, the high blood pressure numbers) and repeatedly exposing their entire body—including the healthy body parts—to the toxins in that pill. Does that sound like effective health care to you?

Here's the bottom line: medicine and surgery can be effective for crisis care. They may help you win a battle, but they will never help you win the war. It's a misnomer to call medicine and surgery a "health-care" system. It is really a "crisis-care" system, and even in a crisis, it doesn't always work! Plus, there are always some negative consequences to medicines that have to be weighed against any supposed positives.

So, if you're blood pressure shoots up to 190/150, then by all means take a blood pressure–lowering medication. But after you pop that pill, it's up to you to determine why the blood pressure is high and do something about it so that you can get off the drugs and be healthy again!

> "If you want health, wealth, and prosperity, you need to do the exact opposite of what everyone else is doing."

Maximized Living Drug Policy

Through endless reports on the serious and often deadly side effects of ALL medications from aspirin to antidepressants and everything in between, you should be aware of the dangers of taking either prescription or over-the-counter medications. Clearly, you should know to think twice when someone tells you to "take two and call me in the morning." However, only your medical doctor can prescribe drugs or tell you to get off of drugs. *That's the practice of medicine.*

Through Maximized Living, we want to make you aware of the hazards of poor lifestyle decisions while helping you to create optimum function and healing in your body. This is done through the Five Essentials of Maximized Living.

MaximizedLivingMakeover.com

CRISIS CARE

Watch this special video from Dr. Ben Lerner on Zone 2 vs. Zone 1 living.

In time, you must begin to judge for yourself whether your medications are keeping you alive, merely palliating symptoms of an unhealthy body, or actually causing some of the ailments you suffer from. The bottom line is that taking any drugs will cause some level of adverse side effects. With the guidance of your prescribing physician, you need to make your own best decisions on medication. As you heal, work with your medical doctors to help you reduce or eliminate the drugs you're on.

If you are relying on medicine or surgery to give you long-term health or pain relief, then you have fallen victim to the flawed medical model. It won't work. But there is something that will work, and it's much closer than you might think! There are five essential steps to Maximized Living, and if you follow these five steps, you will be able to achieve a level of energy, health, and overall well-being that you may never have experienced before. Let's now look at the five essentials needed for living to that potential.

TAKE A STEP FORWARD!

Your body is an amazing, self-healing machine. It doesn't need any help to heal—it just needs a lack of interference. Once you get out of the way of your body's natural healing processes, your body is programmed to do the rest.

1. Be sure to watch the special video on the body's self-healing properties—it's on the website. And while you're there, use the online BMI (Body Mass Index) calculator (there's also an explanation of what BMI is) and learn more about your body type.

2. Health is when all the cells of the body are functioning and healing at 100 percent. It's not the absence of symptoms. As with heart disease, sometimes the first "symptom" that you have it is sudden death. This was the case with Dr. Ben Lerner's father. If you haven't already been to the website to watch his moving account of this experience, be sure to go today.

3. Five out of six Americans will die from a degenerative disease, and the vast majority of the time the disease is the fault of the person who is degenerating. This isn't insensitive or mean—it is filled with hope for you! If degenerative disease is something we cause by our lifestyle, then that also means that it's something you can avoid by changing your lifestyle, starting today.

4. One of the leading causes of death is modern medicine. We're not referring to mistakes like cutting off the wrong leg, being injected with the wrong drug, or getting ten times the prescribed dose. We're talking about people getting the right procedure, for the right problem, in the right way, at the right time, in the right dose—and dying. That's why medical doctors are terrified of being patients. Modern medicine is useful for crisis care—but it's much better to avoid the crisis in the first place. That's why the Five Essentials of Maximized Living are vital—they help keep you out of crisis!

5. It is vital to change how you think about health. Maximized Living comes when you focus on *establishing health* instead of *treating symptoms*. When you merely treat symptoms, you almost never address the underlying problem. For instance, headaches aren't caused by aspirin deficiencies—but they are caused by something. Aspiring may make the pain the go away for a few hours, but it won't solve what's causing the pain—and neither will you, because you're focused on the symptom. The Five Essentials of Maximized Living are the key to establishing health, creating the environment for your body to heal itself, and removing the actual cause of the symptoms. If you haven't already watched the video about finding the cause for symptoms, go to www.MaximizedLivingMakeover.com

> The "medical model" is responsible for over one million deaths per year.

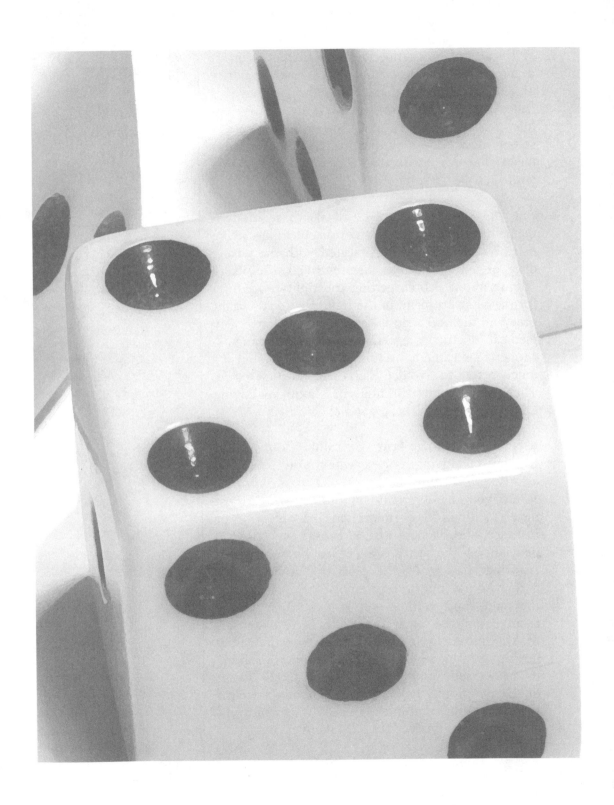

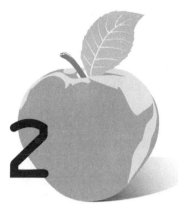

2

The Five Essentials: What Are They and Why Do They Matter to Me?

There are five essentials to maximized living. They are called essentials because each one is absolutely necessary to live the full, healthy life you were intended to live. These are five essentials that are the irreducible minimums (meaning that you need to do these five things if you do nothing else!) to keep the cells in your body in top shape and replicating normally for optimal body function. They are physical laws of the universe.

Many would attempt to dilute health down to only one discipline or essential, and that's, "It's all about nutrition." Nothing, however, could be farther from the truth. Yes, it is important to eat well, but if you ignore the other four components of maximized living, your body will not even assimilate the good food you have eaten. Yes, it is wonderful to get in great physical shape, but if you ignore the other essentials, you may end up a miserable, albeit muscular person who will look great in a coffin someday but who failed to experience fulfilling relationships.

To function and heal normally; to experience your health potential; and to lead a long, joyful, fulfilling life,

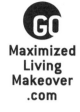

Maximized Living Makeover .com

MaximizedLivingMakeover.com

PRACTICE—NOT PERFECT!

Read a special report from Dr. Greg Loman on how striving for perfection can actually be a barrier to maximized living, and how steady, small improvements can make all the difference to experience and sustain maximized living.

> The five essentials are the irreducible minimums that you need to do if you do nothing else!

MaximizedLivingMakeover.com

MAXIMIZED LIVING SYNERGY

Read a special report from Dr. Charles Majors on how each area of maximized living affects the others—and how they all work together to help you achieve incredible health and happiness.

MaximizedLivingMakeover.com

FIVE ESSENTIALS

Take a test to determine your level of proficiency with the five Essentials.

MaximizedLivingMakeover.com

STATINS

They're prescribed like Life Savers, but are they right for you? Learn what statins are, what they do, and the latest ones to be recalled.

you must address all of the five essentials—every single one. It's not about perfecting all five, because health-food nuts, superior athletes, and stress gurus don't necessarily live better, longer lives. It's about consciously paying attention to and trying to live by the principles of the five essentials. When you practice them, you give yourself the best chance to experience what all of us want out of our bodies and our lives—life to the max!

What Are the Five Essentials?

After years of research, study, and treating people of all ages, shapes, and sizes, the five essentials we have discovered that people must practice in order to achieve long, satisfying, healthy maximized lives are the following:

ESSENTIAL 1:	Minimize the use of drugs, other toxins, and surgery.
ESSENTIAL 2:	Maximize nerve supply.
ESSENTIAL 3:	Maximize quality nutrition.
ESSENTIAL 4:	Maximize oxygen and lean muscle.
ESSENTIAL 5:	Maximize peace and strong relationships.

While most of these may seem commonsensical at first glance, it is amazing how many of us do not practice any— let alone all—of the five essentials on a regular, daily basis. We say we want to eat well, but do we understand what that really means? What "good" foods really are? We take deep breaths and exercise when we can, but do we know the best ways to get oxygen deep into our tissues and the right ways to build muscles so that they keep our body running at its peak? If we answer honestly, most of us don't—and if we don't know how to live those two essentials well, chances are good that we don't fully understand how the other three can benefit us either.

Let's take a look at why the five essentials are so crucial to our overall well being and how they work with each other to produce maximized lives:

How Do the Essentials Work?

There is only one way to well-being. It's not treatment; it's care. Taking care of yourself (with doctors helping you with this care) by removing components of your lifestyle that are out of alignment with how the body works and by eliminating what goes in your body that interferes goes hand in hand with the five essentials.

Take, for example, the enormous eruption of depression and now the backlash created by treating it with antidepressant drugs. The truth is, that condition, along with most others, is a complex problem brought on by issues with body function and lifestyle. Quick fixes like toxic, mind-altering drugs are not the best answer. Depression and anxiety have been found to be associated with multiple causes—not just one. To get well, the causes—not just the symptoms—must be addressed. While there are rare cases of actual organic issues with the brain, the large majority of those with depression suffer from the effects of modern lifestyle on the brain and emotions.

Here's how interfering with the five essentials plays a major role in developing depression:

Essential 1: Toxicity—Toxins and chemicals found for example in medications and refined foods affect hormone balance and glandular function.

Essential 2: Damage or misalignment of the spine and nervous system—Correcting vertebral alignment and posture has a marked effect on the central nervous system and how well it functions and produces well-balanced body chemistry.

Essential 3: Poor Nutrition
  • Diets high in carbohydrates leave a constant level of insulin in the system, which lowers serotonin levels and causes inflammation.

ESPECIALLY FOR THE YOUNG, FABULOUS, AND SYMPTOM FREE

Dr. Ben Lerner reports on how a lack of symptoms doesn't mean lack of disease. For many people who die of heart attacks, their first symptom is death.

Consciously pay attention to and try to live by the principles of the Five Essentials.

It is important to eat well, but if you ignore the other four components, your body will not even assimilate the good food you have eaten.

MaximizedLivingMakeover.com

WATER

View a special report on water from Dr. Charles Majors. There's reverse-osmosis water, oxygenated water, distilled water, spring water, bottled water, filtered water, and plain old tap water. Discover the best kind for you and your family.

> When you practice the five essentials, you give yourself the best chance to experience what all of us want—life to the max!

- Imbalances in omega-3 and omega-6 ratios have been found to be the first factor to address regarding depression, according to professors at Harvard and Oxford universities.
- pH balance that is off can lead to inflammation. Stimulants, sugars, and artificial additives negatively affect brain function.
- Nutrient deficiency can be solved by food and supplementation.

Essential 4: Sedentary lifestyle—Inactivity and a lack of intentional exercise has many damaging effects to function and mental health. That's why exercise consistently matches or exceeds the benefits of antidepressants.

Essential 5: Lack of sleep, poor time management, and stress—Identifying and resolving the effects of inadequate sleep, abundant stress, and negative attitude will slow down the neurotransmitter burnout these issues cause.

Other Modern Conditions

Most, if not all, modern conditions—from pain syndromes and cancer to heart disease and degenerative illness—can be addressed through maximized living. It's a natural way of living that is best prescribed long before the conditions arise in the first place and must be applied that much more once the symptoms show up.

The major health issue of high cholesterol can be held up to the five essentials in the same way. Rather then utilizing dangerous, controversial statins, there are other solutions to look at.

Maximized Living Solution

Essential 1: Avoid modern "nutrition": flour, sugar, fried foods.

Essential 2: Improve liver and bowel function.

Essential 3: Embrace proper nutrition: a diet robust in soluble fiber.

Essential 4: Improve fat to muscle ratios.

Essential 5: Reduce stress levels, which create an inflammatory response *requiring* an increase in cholesterol levels to protect, heal, and repair nerve tissue.

MaximizedLivingMakeover.com

DEPRESSION

Depression is the battleground on the road to maximized living. Learn in depth about how the five Essentials can help you start to feel better—and live better—right now. View a special report by Dr. Greg Loman about antidepressants and the five Essentials.

Here's a good example of what happens when the five essentials are not put into practice.

Joan Smith is a thirty-eight-year-old secretary for a medium-sized law firm. She is married with two kids at home, ages nine and eleven. Joan wakes at 6:00 a.m., gets the kids going, and heads out of the house by 7:30 a.m. to get the kids to school and get to work by 8:00 a.m. She typically grabs breakfast on the run—coffee with artificial sweetener and bagel with cream cheese—eats lunch at her desk or out with colleagues, and rushes out of the office at 4:30 p.m. to pick the kids up from after-school care, and gets home each night to fix dinner for her family. A typical dinner might consist of roasted chicken; some kind of frozen green vegetable or salad from a bag; rice or stuffing from a box; and a dessert of ice cream or prepackaged cookies.

Joan works forty hours a week, volunteers at her son's school, goes to church on Sunday mornings, and helps her kids with their homework after dinner each weeknight, in between loads of laundry. She connects with her husband, John, for conversation or television watching after 9:30 p.m. when the kids go to bed and before John's head hits the pillow around 11:00 p.m. Then she folds the last load

Identifying and resolving the effects of inadequate sleep, abundant stress, and negative attitude will slow down the neurotransmitter burnout these issues cause.

---

of laundry or straightens the kitchen, reads a few pages of a novel, and goes to sleep around midnight.

On the weekends, the family tries to do something together on Friday nights, heads to the kids' sports activities on Saturdays, and on Saturday nights sees friends, or John and Joan try to have a "date night." Sundays are taken up by church, lunch, homework, and getting groceries or other needed supplies before the work and school week starts again.

Joan often feels tired, stressed, and overwhelmed. Her back hurts from leaning over her desk to see the computer, and her neck hurts from leaning her head to the side to hold the phone between her ear and shoulder so she can type while she talks. She hasn't been to a doctor in years. She pops an aspirin or ibuprofen when her headaches and backaches get too intense and an antacid when her stomach acts up.

Her relationship with John is often tense, and she never feels like she is giving enough to her husband or kids—let alone finding any time for herself. She would love to exercise more and knows she isn't always eating right, but doesn't know how or when to fit it all in. After years of this lifestyle, Joan finds herself experiencing depression and eventually feels like she is having a breakdown. She finally sees a doctor who prescribes antianxiety drugs and antidepressants.

If you asked Joan if she was living a maximized life, she'd probably laugh in your face—or break down and cry.

Joan Smith is most likely just like you, sprinting through life, skipping essentials of well-being, ignoring the symptoms of degeneration as they pop up, and eventually using drugs to get through your day. If you're saying that's not you, it most likely eventually will be. Most of us are part of the DA club—Degenerators Anonymous—living lives that cause us to deteriorate physically and mentally until there is nothing left.

But there is hope. By applying the five essentials to your everyday life, you can make vast improvements in your health, wealth, happiness, and life. In each of the next five chapters, we will take an in-depth look at each of the five essentials and what they can mean to your life. So what are you waiting for? It's time to regenerate through maximized living!

TAKE A STEP FORWARD!

The Five Essentials of Maximized Living are:
1. Minimize the use of drugs, other toxins, and surgery.
2. Maximize nerve supply.
3. Maximize quality nutrition.
4. Maximize oxygen and lean muscle.
5. Maximize peace and strong relationships.

1. Remember that each of the Essentials is important—none of them are optional. If you're consumed by worry, it doesn't matter how much you exercise or eat right—the stress will kill you long before degeneration has a chance to get to you. If you're taking a prescription medicine that should have never been approved in the first place, it can cause damage, disease, or even death—regardless of how much peace you have in your life. And if your brain isn't communicating with the rest of your body, your health can be interrupted in a moment—just ask anyone suffering from the effects of a car wreck.

2. Remember that all of the Essentials work together. For example, stressed out people tend to sleep less—and eat more. So it's easier to eat well when you're experiencing maximum peace. By the same token, your body gives off endorphins after you exercise, which enhances your feelings of peace. And eating the right foods at the right times keeps your blood sugar where it needs to be, which gives you consistent energy throughout the day, allowing you to be at your very best from the time you get up in the morning until the time you go bed.

3. All of us naturally do better in some of the Essentials more than others. One of the great benefits at www.MaximizedLivingMakeover.com is that it allows you to get extra help and targeted insight in those areas that are most challenging to you. Get familiar with it today, so you can quickly find resources and the help you need on this journey.

MaximizedLivingMakeover.com

DEGENERATORS ANONYMOUS:

Identify your number-one struggle, and get practical, specific advice on positive steps you can take today for

Energy level
Stress level
Physical well being
Feeling of well being
Stress
Obesity
Anorexia
Diet
Exercise
Relationships
Depression
Anxiety
Being overwhelmed
Chronic pain
Cancer
Heart disease
Diabetes
Depression
ADD or ADHD

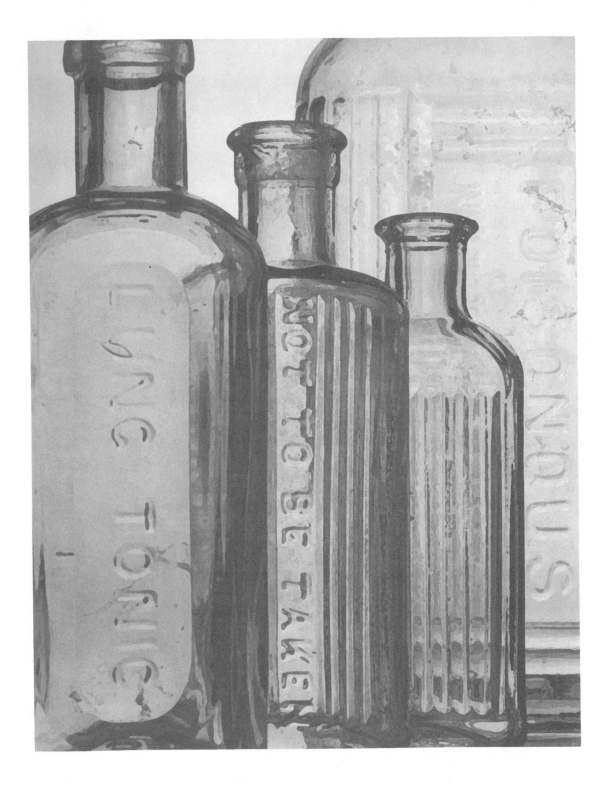

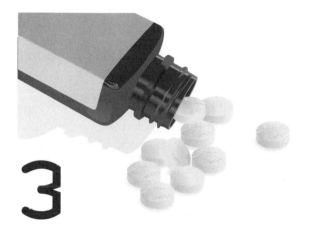

3

ESSENTIAL 1:
Minimize the Use of Drugs, Other Toxins, and Surgery

How many prescription drugs do you take each year? Would it surprise you to know that nearly four billion prescription drugs are ingested in the United States annually, and more than seventy thousand chemicals are used commercially? Additionally, more than three thousand chemicals are added to our food supply, and over ten thousand are used in food processing, preserving, and storage. That's a lot of chemicals— literally tons and tons of chemicals! It's also a lot of toxicity that finds its way, accidentally and on purpose, into our bodies every day. *Bottom line: We are being poisoned—and we are giving the poison to ourselves.*

Toxicity in the United States—and moving abroad as other countries adopt America's health-care model—has reached catastrophic and historic levels. Over the past century we have grown sadly accustomed to the growing number of heart attacks and cancer cases, but today we can also add to the list increases in many other diseases.

Back in 1970, only 4 in 10,000 children developed autism,[5] a brain and immune system disorder that usually develops between birth and age six. In February 2007, the

Go
Maximized Living Makeover .com

MaximizedLivingMakeover.com

AUTISM
The epidemic the medical community won't acknowledge. With tens of thousands of parents convinced that vaccinations have harmed their children and the medical authorities flatly denying it, you need to watch this special report by Dr. Charles Majors on the exploding rate of autism in the United States and what can be done through detoxification and supplementation.

> We are being poisoned—and we are giving the poison to ourselves.

MaximizedLivingMakeover.com

CHRONIC FATIGUE
View a special report from Dr. Ben Lerner on chronic fatigue and fibromyalgia, with critical information on detoxification and supplementation.

> Toxicity in the United States has reached catastrophic and historic levels.

Centers for Disease Control published an analysis of 2002 data which revealed 1 in 94 to 1 in 303 American children in 2002 developed autism by age eight.[6] That's a national average of 1 child in every 150 or more suffering from Autism Spectrum Disorders (ASDs).[7]

And that's not all. One in three adults develops autoimmune diseases like multiple sclerosis, rheumatoid arthritis, and lupus, a disability in which the body's immune system starts to attack itself. In fact, America has more degenerative diseases like heart disease, cancer, arthritis, diabetes, and Alzheimer's than any other country in the world. (Although other countries are catching "down" to us as they adopt our health-care model.)

Even more startling and puzzling to doctors are the numbers of people suffering from mysterious illnesses such as chronic fatigue syndrome and fibromyalgia. Now add on the new or constantly increasing presence of diseases and disorders like attention deficit disorder and attention deficit hyperactivity disorder (in both children and adults), asthma (which has increased in children more than ten times in the last decade), reflux, thyroid failure, Parkinson's, and so many others. We have to ask ourselves: "What on earth is going on, and how can we stop the madness?"

Answer: We can choose to follow Essential 1 and stop poisoning ourselves.

Today, your family's ability to remain healthy, avoid suffering, and prevent disease is not as simple as eating the perfect diet and exercising. It is also not as simple as taking prescribed drugs for whatever seems to be ailing you. On the contrary, if we don't accept Essential 1 and acknowledge the constant invasion of toxic substances and poisonous buildup in our bodies, it will be impossible to avoid the disease onslaught this new millennium has been providing.

Medication—The Number-One Cause of Toxicity

Healthy lifestyles are the biggest threat to the growth and expansion of the drug industry and its consequences in our society. A recent *Forbes* magazine cover article, "Pharma's New Enemy: Clean Living," thoroughly addressed this subject from the position of the consumer as well as from the position of the investor. Consider the following perspective from the article:

"Do you really need all those prescription and over the counter pills you are popping? Maybe not. There's a backlash building against the cost, risk and side effects of medication, and it's bad news for the pharmaceutical industry."

The message was driven home even more powerfully when the article noted:

"The results of pill dependence are insidious and devastating: billions of dollars in ever higher drug costs; millions of people enduring sometimes highly toxic side-effects; and close to 2 million cases each year of drug complications that result in 180,000 deaths of life-threatening illnesses in the elderly."[8]

As the article notes, "Every few years the ultimate medical catastrophe: a miracle cure that turns out to be toxic." (Think Vioxx, Avandia, hormone replacement therapy, Paxil, and the like.) Every drug is a toxin! It used to be that an apple a day would keep the doctor away. Nowadays, the recommendation is an aspirin a day. Well, it turns out that an aspirin a day for at least five years increases a woman's chance of developing breast cancer by 80 percent compared to nonregular aspirin users. If I were you, I'd take my chances with the apple.

And if you get breast cancer, chances are the drugs prescribed for that cause more harm than good. Many women have been prescribed Tamoxifen for the treatment of their breast cancer. Unfortunately, research now shows that taking Tamoxifen increases the chance of incidence and death from *uterine* cancer[9].

Even something as seemingly harmless as over-the-counter children's cough medicine can be deadly. A cough rarely kills a child, but cough medicine and cough syrup just might. The Centers for Disease Control recently released a warning to parents after more than 1,500 infants and toddlers wound up in emergency rooms and 3 children

MaximizedLivingMakeover.com

CHOLESTEROL

Masking the symptoms is not the same as curing them. Watch a special report by Dr. Charles Majors on a prescription drug that lowers cholesterol but not the risk of dying of a heart attack or stroke, and introduces a host of dangerous side effects.

America has more degenerative diseases like heart disease, cancer, arthritis, diabetes, and Alzheimer's than any other country in the world.

COLD, FLU, OR EAR INFECTIONS

What do you do when your child has the cold, flu, or ear infection? Read this special report by Dr. Greg Loman about how you can dramatically reduce the incidence of your child contracting these diseases in the first place.

If we don't acknowledge the constant invasion of toxic substances and poisonous buildup in our bodies, it will be impossible to avoid disease onslaught.

---

died because of reactions or overdoses of pediatric cold medicines. Behind the scenes, one doctor admitted, "fluids and patience are the best treatment."

The most common prescription drugs sold in the U.S. today, and possibly the most toxic to your system, are antidepressant medications. Symptoms resulting from a negative reaction to an antidepressant drug easily can be mistaken for a comorbid psychiatric disorder such as anxiety, bipolar illness, obsessive-compulsive disorder, or schizophrenia. Clinical guidelines indicate that these disorders also require pharmacologic intervention. If more drugs are added to already toxic brain chemistry, it can result in the exacerbation of life-threatening symptoms and rapid clinical deterioration of the person's mental status. Any drug that induces hallucinations, mania, or psychotic behavior should be discontinued immediately. Antipsychotic drugs should never be added when symptoms are a direct result of drug toxicity.

While antidepressants are the most common prescription drugs, the most commonly administered drugs are vaccinations, "preventive" measures injected or swallowed in a cocktail of toxins. Barbara Loe Fisher of the National Vaccine Institute says vaccines contain a variety of harmful substances:

> *"Vaccines can contain formaldehyde, phenoxyethanol, gluteraldehyde, sodium chloride, MSG, gelatin, hydrochloric acid, sodium acetate, hydrogen peroxide, yeast protein, lab-altered viruses and bacteria and unidentified contaminants...*[10]
> *There is more mercury in a flu shot than can be legally disposed of in most city garbage dumps...*[11]
> *A two-month old baby can be injected with four times the amount of aluminum in vaccines on one day than is considered safe."*[12]

As the parent of a DPT vaccine–injured child, Fisher cofounded the nonprofit National Vaccine Information Center in 1982 to prevent vaccine injuries and deaths through public education. Back then, Fisher notes that pediatricians were giving children twenty-three doses of seven vaccines, including vaccines for measles, mumps, and rubella.[13]

By 2007, the numbers of doses of vaccines the federal government recommended for universal use by the age of twelve had more than doubled to fifty-four doses of sixteen vaccines! These include the following: diphtheria (six doses), pertussis (six doses), tetanus (six doses), polio (four doses), measles (two doses), mumps (one dose), rubella (one dose), HIB (four doses), hepatitis B (three doses), chicken pox (two doses), hepatitis A (two doses), pneumococcal (four doses), rotavirus (three doses), influenza (five doses), meningococcal (one dose), and HPV (three doses for girls).[14] This is a radical increase in more toxins than we have been taught to believe are good for us—and for our children!

The Harmful Effects of Surgery

The surgical element of Essential 1 really needs little explanation. Your body was created like a finely made car or watch. There are no extra parts neither should parts be altered. While some may believe or even experience relief from surgery in the short term, by law, you suffer down the road.

Every part in your body is there for a reason and operates as it should, provided you take care of it. Man will never know all of the reasons why the parts are there, as man cannot create another man. Therefore, a human who alters, fuses together, tinkers with, or removes body parts from another human is similar to someone who knows nothing at all about cars or watches altering, fusing, eliminating, or tinkering with their mechanical parts. Poor function, breakdown, or end of lifespan is inevitable.

Everyday Environmental Toxins

In addition to drugs, there are countless chemicals and other toxins we encounter in our environments every day. In the "National Report on Human Exposure to Environmental Chemicals" prepared by the CDC, the study

READ

MaximizedLivingMakeover.com

BLACK-BOX WARNINGS

As if some medicines weren't risky enough, even the medical community gives them the infamous "black-box warning" from the FDA. Read Dr. Greg Loman's research about how to spot these warnings, the common prescriptions that have them, and why the whole concept is so shocking.

It used to be that an apple a day would keep the doctor away. Nowadays, the recommendation is an aspirin a day. I'd take my chances with the apple.

TOXIC TOP TEN

For alternatives to the toxic top ten, learn the latest on the top-rated products.

> The most common prescription drugs sold in the U.S. today and possibly the most toxic to your system are antidepressant medications.

focused on 116 environmental toxins that find their way into the human population through pollution or consumer products. Exposure was measured through the blood and urine samples of a group of volunteers. The report found positive results for 89 chemicals.[15]

These toxins will accumulate in our tissues over time, and this accumulation is what many researchers now believe is the heart of modern-day disease. Columbia University's School of Public Health reported that 95 percent of all cancer is caused by diet and environment, referring to the slow accumulation or stockpiling of chemicals over decades, leading to disease.

Interestingly, our parents, or the generation before us, didn't experience these symptoms until their sixties. The generation that follows ours is experiencing these symptoms in their twenties. In our clinics, we are starting to see teenagers exhibiting degenerative diseases, including these newer types of illnesses like depression, chronic fatigue, fibromyalgia, and hormonally related sickness.

This process of degeneration and toxic accumulation starts even before birth. The toxic intake of the mother and the toxins residing in her body directly affect the fetus. Today, scientists believe that this toxic accumulation is one of the leading causes of birth defects. Beyond the womb, this toxicity continues, and by the age of six some kids have already filled their buckets halfway with cancer-causing chemicals, elements, and toxins.

You can't eliminate all toxins or stress yourself out trying, but you can trust your body to do what it was created to do. When it is working at its optimum level—healing and functioning normally—your body is made to process and remove a certain amount of poison. Not, however, the amounts it has having to deal with in "modern" Western living. Even though chances are good you have been exposed for years to toxins you were not even aware of, it's time to become aware of the "Toxic Top Ten" and eliminate them as much as possible in order to live the principle of Essential 1 of Maximized Living.

The Toxic Top Ten

washing detergents,
or and furniture
ners (especial-
and soaps,
toilet bowl

ling

—found in

free-range
void pork.

nated oils,
fined, fast,
xcitotoxins
amate), as-
hydrolyzed

containing

use extra virgin
oderate heats and
eats to reduce sticking.

eavy metals, contaminants,

urified water.

THINK EATING HEALTHY MEANS EATING EXPENSIVE?

Think again! Read the story of a stay-at-home mother of five on a tight budget who is able to feed her family the maximized living way.

> Your body was created like a finely made car or watch. There are no extra parts neither should parts be altered.

MaximizedLivingMakeover.com

DETOXIFICATION MYTHS VERSUS REALITIES.

You've read about the importance of detoxification, but what's the real story on detoxification? View a special report by Dr. Dan Pompa on the two critical steps for proper detoxification.

> A human who alters, fuses together, tinkers with, or removes body parts from another human is similar to someone who knows nothing at all about cars or watches altering, fusing, eliminating, or tinkering with their mechanical parts.

7. Personal care products—soaps, conditioners, shampoos, toothpaste containing toxic ingredients like Sodium Lauryl Sulfate (SLS), DEA, Propylene Glycol, and fluoride.

    SOLUTION: Use natural products that do not contain these chemicals.

8. Heavy metals: Mercury found in vaccinations, flu shots, silver (amalgam) fillings and fish. Also lead and aluminum found in old paints, toys, and kitchenware.

    SOLUTION: Educate yourself on the ingredients and content of these items and make informed decisions.

9. Biotoxins—Mold and lyme are the most common infiltrators in our homes.

    SOLUTION: These require specialized testing from natural physicians that work specifically in this area.

10. Medicine—The purpose of these volatile chemicals is to radically alter body function and change physiology. They are so toxic that it is a fact that a medicine without a side effect isn't a medicine.

    SOLUTION: Work with your doctors to take as few medications as possible, if any. The obvious solution is Maximized Living.

If you suspect heavy metal or biotoxicity, it is important to be tested and undergo specific treatments designed to remove or neutralize these dangerous, life-ruining poisons. Symptoms of these kinds of poisoning are severe and can include: inability to sleep, fatigue, anxiety, depression, decreased libido, and muscle and joint pain. Go to www.MaximizedLivingMakeover.com to find a specialized provider.

While Essential 1 requires that you minimize (and eliminate, if possible) toxins and other things that can harm your body, the remaining four essentials give you a

... to maximize your body's natural ability ... was created to do—remain healthy and fully ... for life. Through the next four essentials of ...d Living, you'll see a model that makes sense. It ...del you can follow that builds your health up to its ...imum potential rather than treating a condition or a ...isease with manufactured drugs and treatments that do more harm than good.

And if you ever do suffer from a health problem again, what could be a better solution than maximizing your health so that you will not only be symptom free (like a drug or surgery may or may not provide) but also function and heal normally once again? That's maximized living! Let's take a look.

TAKE A STEP FORWARD!

It is vital to stop poisoning yourself! We live in a chemical fog that contaminates the air we breathe, the water we drink, and the foods we eat. Not only can we not escape it in our homes, sometimes it's more toxic inside our homes than outside. No one knows what the long-term effects of all these drugs are on human beings, but we do see alarming outbreaks of new maladies like fibromyalgia and chronic fatigue, and dramatic increases in the incidence of old maladies like autism. That's why it's vital to control and limit—as much as possible—the chemicals that are within you, and the chemicals that surround you.

1. Approach taking any drug with extreme caution. Drugs that seem innocuous may not be. The cough medicines that seem completely benign may end up sending your child to the emergency room, and if the Vioxx debacle teaches us anything, it's that today's wonder drug may be tomorrow's class-action lawsuit—that is, if you're alive to sue. We're not saying to not take medicine, or to stop taking medicine—we're saying to proceed with care and get the facts. Your Maximized Living Doctors and Mentors can help you think through all of the dimensions of this important issue. Make sure you find the one closest to you today!

> Toxins will accumulate in our tissues over time, and this accumulation is what many researchers now believe is the heart of modern day disease.

> The generation before us didn't experience symptoms until their sixties. The generation that follows ours is experiencing symptoms in their twenties.

2. Ordinary household utensils and cleaners need to be carefully considered since they can add to the chemical cocktail in your home. The effects of all these substances mixed together isn't well known, so we recommend finding natural alternatives as much as possible. Check www.MaximizedLivingMakeover.com for the products we recommend—which are the products we expose our own families to and use regularly.

3. If you or your environment have been contaminated, it's important to neutralize the effects as fast as possible. Your Maximized Living Doctor or Mentor can help you evaluate your options.

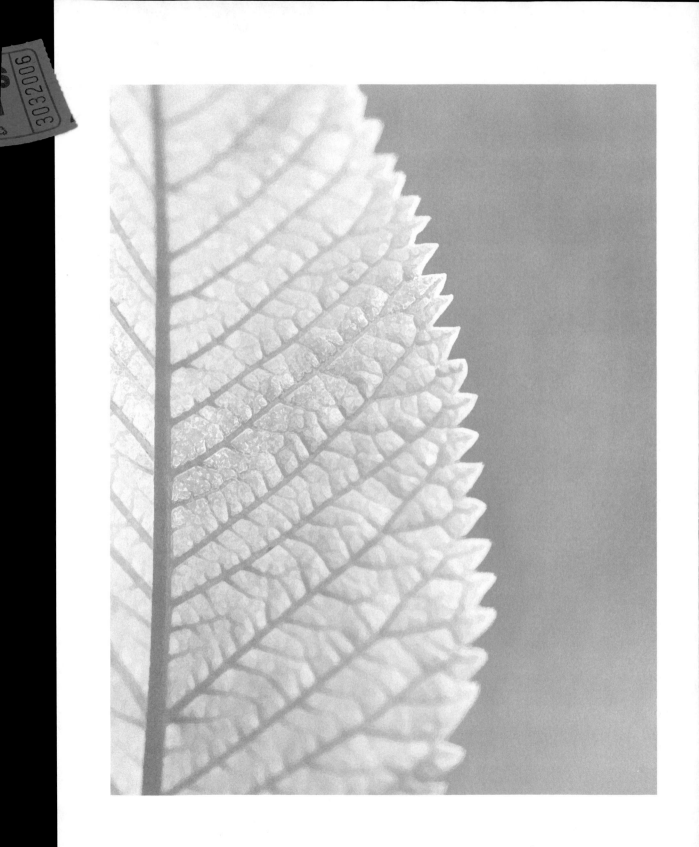

4

ESSENTIAL 2:
Maximized Nerve Supply

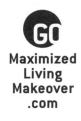

Maximized Living Makeover .com

MaximizedLivingMakeover.com

BACK PAIN

Watch a special video with exercises that are easy to learn to alleviate pain and maximize nerve supply!

When scientists study the development of embryos, they discover that the brain is the first organ to develop. The brain then sends creative power through the spinal cord and nerves to create every cell and organ in your body. (The brain, spinal cord, and nerves make up the central nervous system, the main headquarters of the whole body.) From that first neonatal moment where the brain sends the first impulse down the tiny spinal cord on, that brain power flowing down the spine and nervous system continues to control all function and healing in the body for the rest of your life. Consequently, the spine is your lifeline. All real wellness is ultimately dependent on the spine's and nervous system's ability to provide *maximum nerve supply*.

The central nervous system—the life-power supply—is so powerful and complex that it is able to control millions of cells within dozens of operating systems all at once. This is done without the user even consciously thinking or knowing about it. While the body can go days without water, weeks without food, and minutes without oxygen, it cannot last even a second without the power provided through nerve supply.

> The spine is your lifeline. All real wellness is ultimately dependent on the spine and nervous system's ability to provide *maximum nerve supply*.

MaximizedLivingMakeover.com

FORWARD HEAD SYNDROME

Take the questionnaire to determine if you have Forward Head Syndrome. Learn about the symptoms, dangers, and treatment by Dr. Ben Lerner.

> The body can go days without water, weeks without food, and minutes without oxygen, but cannot last even a second without the power provided through nerve supply.

> Look well to the spine as the cause of disease.
> ~ *Hippocrates, the father of modern medicine*

Ultimately, health, function, and healing are totally controlled by nerve supply. So important are the purveyors of nerve supply that the main organs are encased in their own bony armor. The skull protects the upper brain, and the bones of the spinal column protect the spinal cord and nerve roots.

A common and very likely way to interfere with maximum nerve supply is for the spinal column to become damaged or even shift or rotate out of place. This interference is a major underlying cause of poor physical and emotional health or subpar performance. Yet as important as the spine is, except for the stomach, it's the most regularly abused part of your body. Determining how well your spine is positioned and performing is a major factor in determining whether or not your body is producing a state of health or producing a state of disease.

How do you know if your spine is positioned well and performing correctly? The two primary methods for evaluating proper alignment and position of the spine are posture and x-ray.

Healthy Posture: It's Not Just for Breakfast Anymore

Remember how mothers, especially on TV, used to nag their kids to sit up straight at the breakfast table? That familiar image turns out to contain a lot of wisdom in it. As science continues to reveal, good posture is a major key to good health.

What does good posture look like? When you look at a person from the front, the spine should be straight. The head, shoulders, hips, and feet should be lined up. When you look at a person from the side, the ears should be back over the shoulders and the shoulders should be back over the pelvis.

Posture and spine are abnormal if:

- A person's head is visibly tilted, shifted, or rotated in one direction.
- The head is jutted out in front of the chest and shoulders (forward-head syndrome).
- One hip is higher than the other, turned in one direction, or shifted to one side.
- One shoulder is higher than the other, turned in one direction, or the whole upper body is shifted to one side.

Any time there is abnormal posture, a person's central nervous system is experiencing interference or damage.

> Posture affects and moderates every physical and mental function in the body. Spinal pain, blood pressure, headaches, pulse, lung capacity, and mood are only a small portion of the body's functions that are most easily influenced by posture.
> ~ Dr. C. Norman Shealy, Shealy Institute[16]

X-Ray

The most accurate method for measuring nerve supply—the condition of the spine—is the use of x-rays. When looking at the front view x-ray, the spinal bones (vertebrae) should also be straight. The bones must not be rotated or tilted, and no curvatures to the side (scoliosis) should be present.

The side-view x-ray must reveal three well-placed arcs. The most important arc is in the neck (cervical spine) between the first and last cervical vertebrae (called in medical terminology the C1 and C7). This cervical arc is known as the Arc of Life because life impulses travel directly from the brain down this part of the spinal cord to bring life to the rest of the body. Losing your Arc of Life causes the most severe obstruction to the central nervous system. The other arcs occur in the thoracic (middle) spine and the lumbar (lower) spine.

MaximizedLivingMakeover.com

THE SPINAL CORD
See what parts of your body are controlled by which parts of your spinal cord.

Health, function, and healing are totally controlled by nerve supply.

MaximizedLivingMakeover.com

CHILDREN AND SUBLUXATION

Is your infant or toddler resilient, or do falls and collisions from the early years take a permanent toll on the spine? See a special video on parenting and care for your infant or toddler by Dr. Charles Majors.

> Determining how well your spine is positioned and performing is a major factor in determining whether or not your body is producing a state of health or producing a state of disease.

Vertebral Subluxation
(Misaligned or Dysfunctional Spinal Segment)
The Key Cause of Interference

In popular thinking about wellness, it is understood that poor nutrition, stress, lack of exercise, or a combination of these can interfere with your health and your body's normal function. But spinal interference can actually create a more damaging effect on overall health than the other factors above, since this strikes right at the core of body function. Take, for example, the unfortunate case of the late actor Christopher Reeve. A fall off of a horse jarred his head and caused a vertebra in his upper neck to become fractured and misplaced. As a result, all function in his body was compromised or stopped altogether.

This is a telling example of the horrifying effects of something called *vertebral subluxation*. Vertebral subluxation is any minor or major misalignment of an individual spinal vertebra or several vertebrae (*global subluxation*). These misalignments, which can be so small that they have to be measured with an instrument, invade the spinal cord space, put pressure on the spinal cord, compress nerves, and/or push soft tissue out of the way and into delicate neurological tissue.[17]

Subluxations at the top of the spine, like the one Christopher Reeve suffered, also cause pressure or damage to the brain stem[18]—the area of the nervous system responsible for breathing, heart rate, and many vital automatic functions. The upper cervical spine and brain stem area is so sensitive that Reeve's doctors said you could cover up the damage to his cord and brain stem with the width of the tip of your pinky (approximately one centimeter), yet the damage was so great that Reeve remained a quadriplegic for the rest of his life.

> Vital information travels from the brain and spinal cord to all of the parts of the body. Not only does information travel down the nerve, but also information from the peripheral parts of the body is sent back to the brain and spinal cord at the same time. When this information is interfered with [by vertebral subluxation], a problem arises in the body.
> ~ Dr. Daniel J. Murphy, Neurological Research and Whiplash Expert

MaximizedLivingMakeover.com

HEADACHES

They can seem like a minor nuisance easily treated by aspirin, but your head isn't supposed to hurt. Read this special report by Dr. Greg Loman and learn how to beat the headache habit!

While not all vertebral subluxations cause major paralysis like Reeve suffered, any spinal interference can wreak havoc on your health. Vertebral subluxation and the accompanying poor posture and positive x-ray findings are caused by a number of very common sources:

1. A challenging birth process (particularly one with medical intervention)
2. Falls and collisions as a child
3. Sports injuries
4. Auto accidents and other traumas
5. Poor posture (working in front of a computer, long-distance driving, poor bodily positioning at work, and so forth)
6. Improper sitting and sleeping positions (which includes pillow and mattress problems)
7. Mental stress
8. Chemical stress (Chemical stress is caused by breaking essential 1—ingesting processed foods, medications, and other toxins.)
9. Lack of exercise, which causes a person to have weak or tight muscles

Because most people experience at least one, if not many, of the causes listed above, the presence of spinal misalignment (vertebral subluxation) is epidemic. The longer subluxation exists, the more degeneration and damage there is to the spine and sensitive central nervous system and the organs they control.[19]

No wonder so many people over the age of forty have severe spine, joint, and organ problems. Many of these

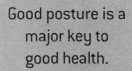

Good posture is a major key to good health.

degenerative conditions eventually require surgery, and millions of people spend their later years dependent on canes, walkers, wheelchairs, adult diapers, and the goodwill of others.

In fact, a shocking 2004 study in the *Journal of the American Geriatrics Society* revealed that mortality could be *predicted* by the spine if it had subluxated to the point where there was an accentuation of the hump in the back called "hyperkyphosis." An elite group of medical scientists found that as the curve in the middle back, the kyphosis, became greater than normal, death came sooner.[20]

Another groundbreaking study published in the medical journal *Spine* again shows the vital, urgent need for normal spinal position. Doctors found that progressive kyphosis of the cervical spine (a loss or reversing of the neck's curve) resulted in destruction of nerve fibers due to chronic compression of the spinal cord similar to what happens with multiple sclerosis.[21]

Hyperkyphosis of your mid back and kyphosis of your neck are easily detectable through posture and x-ray. Hyperkyphosis is typical, although not normal, "old-person posture"—bent over. Kyphosis of the neck is forward-head syndrome. The head is jutted way out in front of the chest typically due to a past auto accident or excessive time in front of the computer or handheld video game system. Both are deadly problems.

In his numerous books written for authorities such as the American Medical Association (AMA), Dr. Rene Cailliet, director of the Department of Physical Medicine and Rehabilitation at the University of Southern California, showed in detail how these spinal problems cause pain, illness, and a quickening of the aging process. Here are just a few of the consequences Dr. Cailliet found:

1. Incorrect head position leads to improper spinal function. It is a major and complex form of vertebral subluxation.
2. The head in forward posture can add up to thirty pounds of abnormal leverage on the cervical spine.

Any time there is abnormal posture, a person's central nervous system is experiencing interference or damage.

3. Forward-head posture results in loss of lung capacity, as it depletes it by as much as 30 percent. This loss of lung capacity leads to heart and blood (vascular) problems. (Here's a quick way to see what we mean: Jut your chin out and flex your head down and try to breathe. You can barely do it. Then tuck your chin in and extend your head backwards. Now you can really fill your lungs.)

4. The entire gastrointestinal system is affected by spinal interference, particularly the large intestine. Loss of good bowel peristaltic function and evacuation is common to forward-head posture and loss of spinal curve.

5. Forward-head posture causes an increase in discomfort and pain. Freedom of motion in the first four cervical vertebrae is a major source of stimuli that causes production of endorphins, the hormones that reduce pain and affect emotions. As a result of this loss of endorphins, many otherwise non-painful sensations are experienced as pain.

6. Forward head posture causes loss of healthy spine-body motion. The entire body becomes rigid as the range of motion becomes diminished. A person's body becomes hunched.

Still other studies reveal that misalignment of the top vertebra of the neck is a key cause of SIDS (sudden infant death syndrome)[22] and that loss of height as an adult of more than 3 centimeters leads to bone loss and radically increases your chance of illness and death.

All of these studies—and the devastating effects on your body as outlined on these pages—show how vital it is to care for your spine. Only with a healthy spine can your body allow for maximum nerve supply, and this is crucial from birth until the last day of your life. A healthy spine pays off in both quality and length of life.

Who knows if the outcome might have been different for Christopher Reeve and the thousands like him if there had been normal spinal alignment prior to their accidents, and

MaximizedLivingMakeover.com

CHIROPRACTICS

Watch Dr. Charles Majors giving a correct chiropractic adjustment.

> Spinal interference damages overall since it strikes right at the core of body function.

Any spinal
interference can
wreak havoc on
your health.

if the maximum ability to absorb forces existed? Potentially, these incidents could have gone from deadly events to just another fall or less devastating injury. Addressing spinal health prior to problems gives you your best chance for wellness, prevention, and safety.

The Spine-Brain Connection

With the ability to measure brain activity and its connection to physical health improving each year, studies and theories on the brain-body connection are becoming more and more popular. The more we discover about the functions of the brain and the pathways through which it communicates with our cells and senses, the more likely we are to expand our mental, emotional, and functional capacities and overcome disease.

With so much emphasis on the brain-body connection and how the brain keeps the body going, a logical question must be asked: What keeps the brain going? Paradoxically, the answer to this question is simply *the body*. While the brain is keeping the body healing and vibrating along, nutrients from eating, drinking, breathing, and the products of cellular function keep the brain healing and vibrating.

Nutrients essential to the brain for survival—such as oxygen, glucose, and others—are transported from the body to the brain through the fluid that flows inside your spinal canal. This fluid is called the cerebrospinal (brain-spine) fluid or CSF. This fluid gets from the spine to brain with the use of a CSF pump. This CSF pump doesn't use electricity. The power for the pump is generated by movement of the sacrum (lowest portion of the spine) and the cervical spine (upper portion of the spine).

In order for the CSF pump to move effectively, you need a healthy spinal column. Irregular or reduced motion of the sacrum and/or cervical spine due to vertebral subluxation in either of these areas will lead to abnormal and reduced flow of oxygen, glucose, and other important nutrients to the brain. That is why the spine-brain connection is so important. A bad back or a bad neck will literally give you a bad brain.[23] A healthy spine, therefore, not only gets you functioning better, but also it gets you thinking clearer.

Proof of the life-saving, life-extending benefits of attaining and maintaining maximum nerve supply showed up in a virtual "Fountain of Youth" study at the University of Lund. Researchers took patients who had taken some care of their spine through visiting a chiropractor a few times and compared them to those that had been taking care of their spine and nerve supply for a long period of time. In these two groups, the researchers checked to see how well they dealt with oxidative stress—a key variable in aging and the development of disease.

Simply stated, as we live life, we are subjected to physical, biochemical, and psychological stress. Our ability to repair damaged DNA is an important factor in health and longevity. Oxidative stress is now a broadly accepted theory of how we age and develop disease. Oxidative stress results in DNA damage, and it inhibits DNA repair. The people that had been under long-term chiropractic care of their spine showed far greater ability to resist DNA damage and to repair damage that was done.[24]

Now that you fully understand how crucial it is to take care of your spine every day of your life, how do you do it? How does a person maximize nerve supply and minimize vertebral subluxation—in order to gain maximized living? It's not as difficult as you might think.

Taking Care of Your Spine— Maximizing Nerve Supply

The best way to maintain proper care of your spine and minimize, if not eliminate, vertebral subluxation is to receive chiropractic care regularly. Even though many people still believe that chiropractic adjustments are little more than "hocus pocus," today's research proves beyond the shadow of a doubt how mistaken that belief is.

Among scientists, it's commonly understood that you can't prove, disprove, or improve anything that you can't measure. Today, nutritionists, exercise physiologists, and chiropractors have the means to measure their results.

MaximizedLivingMakeover.com

SCOLIOSIS
Read a special report from Dr. Ben Lerner on a safe and surgery-free way to treat this dangerous condition.

The presence of spinal misalignment is epidemic. The longer it exists, the more degeneration and damage there is.

Only with a healthy spine can your body allow for maximum nerve supply.

SLIPPED OR
RUPTURED DISKS
Nonsurgical solutions to this
common debilitating condition.

> Addressing
> spinal health
> prior to problems
> gives you your
> best chance
> for wellness,
> prevention, and
> safety.

> The brain keeps
> the body healing
> and nutrients from
> eating, drinking,
> breathing, and the
> products of cellular
> function keep the
> brain healing.

Chiropractors, in particular, have taken the best of what neurological and chiropractic research has to offer and combined it to discover even more about what a healthy spine should look like and what can be done to treat the unhealthy spine than has ever been known before.

Chiropractic is based on the accurate and specific measurement of the spine, particularly the upper cervical spine, which houses the lower brain and most of the vital parts of the spinal cord. Newer research on the brain and nervous system, as well as ever-advancing methods for measuring the normal alignment of the healthy spine, has built upon that foundation to bring the science of chiropractic to an unmatched cutting-edge level in today's wellness world.

Based on neurological research, the laws of physics, engineering, mathematics, and endless studies of the spine, doctors, scientists, and researchers of all kinds have developed an optimum model of the upright spine. These models have been published in the world's most prestigious medical journals. We can now distinguish a normal, healthy spine and nervous system from an abnormal, unhealthy one using measurable factors. Just as we know normal, healthy blood pressure or cholesterol ranges, we now know normal, healthy spinal ranges as well as abnormal, unhealthy ones. A chiropractor can attain precise measurements of your spine, make an accurate assessment of the damage to your spine and nervous system, make equally accurate recommendations for care or rehabilitation and determine a clear-cut prognosis.

In addition to using the spinal x-rays and examination of the patient's posture to evaluate spine and nervous-system health, advances in technology have brought tests like EMG (electromyography, which records the electrical activity of muscles) and computerized range of motion and muscle evaluations to give even more insight into the presence of neurological interference, abnormal spinal alignment, malposition of the spinal curves, joint degeneration, and other parts of the vertebral subluxation complex.

What all this means is that the best—and safest—way to take care of your spine is by receiving chiropractic adjustments. One of the great medical myths about chiropractic adjustments is that most people think it is merely some sort of "popping" of the neck or "twisting and cracking" of the back—not unlike popping your own neck or twisting and cracking your spouse's back when he or she feels tight after work.

The truth about a chiropractic adjustment is that there are dozens of ways to analyze vertebral subluxation and more than a hundred ways to adjust and correct spinal problems. There are light-touch adjustments, small and large instrument adjustments, adjustments using trigger points and reflexes, adjustments using specialized tables, multiple forms of hand-only adjustments, as well as techniques that focus on only certain areas of the spine. Vastly dissimilar to manipulations performed by osteopaths and physical therapists, specific, scientific chiropractic adjustments are not generalized mobilizations of the spine. Rather, using various methods of evaluation, chiropractors actually use precise contact points designed to gently shift an individual segment or segments of the spine and extremities in a very specific direction.

And unlike many medical procedures, chiropractic adjustments are incredibly safe. In a study reported in *Spine Medical Journal* in October 2007 of more than 19,700 patients who underwent more than 50,000 cervical spine adjustments, a team of researchers concluded that the risk of having a serious adverse event from "getting your neck cracked" is none. (The manipulation technique at the focus of this safety study was defined as the application of high-velocity/low-amplitude or mechanically assisted thrust to the cervical spine.) Patients were followed, and any adverse symptoms recorded immediately, and up to seven days after treatment. *There were no reports of serious adverse events.*[25]

In comparison, the chance of serious adverse events in hospitals (traditional medical treatment) is 1.5 million per year, with a cost of $3.5 billion.[26]

MaximizedLivingMakeover.com

NERVE SUPPLY
Learn more about the connection between maximum nerve supply and the symptoms associated with perimenopause and menopause.

A bad back or a bad neck will give you a bad brain. A healthy spine gets you functioning better and thinking clearer.

The best way to maintain proper care of your spine and minimize, if not eliminate, vertebral subluxation is to receive chiropractic care regularly.

50 THE NEW 30

Fifty really can be the new thirty, provided you take proper care of your spine! Read a special report by Dr. Ben Lerner on spinal hygiene for those committed to enjoying life!

If you want a practical proof of chiropractic safety: Malpractice insurance carriers do not use myth or bias to determine their premiums. They use raw data based on the likelihood that a doctor would injure someone and be sued. While medical professionals can pay a hundred thousand dollars per year or more for their malpractice coverage, chiropractors pay barely a fraction of this, with premiums as low as only a few hundred dollars per year.

Two Additional Ways to Care for Your Spine

1. Therapeutic reconstructive care—With many spinal problems, including complications such as forward-head syndrome, disc degeneration, osteoarthritis, scoliosis, and loss of normal curves, certain additional spinal care techniques need to be applied in addition to chiropractic adjustments. Therapeutic and reconstructive treatment seeks to rebuild what might be lost, and includes:

- Stretching and weights used to correct the position of the skull (eliminate forward-head syndrome) and restore or increase the curves in the neck (Arc of Life) and upper and lower back.

- Strengthening the musculature in the back of the neck and upper shoulders to hold the head, neck, and upper spine in a normal position.

- Stretching, exercising, and blocking to correct imbalances in posture and lateral curvatures (scoliosis).

- The use of specific chiropractic equipment for the rehydrating of discs and the regenerating of bone.

A chiropractor can attain precise measurements of your spine, make an accurate assessment, make equally accurate recommendations and determine a clear-cut prognosis.

⚡Note: Only highly trained chiropractors can offer these treatments. Standard manipulation, exercise, and physical therapy will not resolve forward-head posture, scoliosis, disc degeneration, or arthritis. Neither will taking medications or having surgery for the resulting effects of these conditions.

2. Spinal hygiene—There was a time when nearly everyone over the age of forty had false teeth—or needed them. Fortunately, Timmy the Tooth and hundreds of other consumer awareness campaigns led by the American Dental Association showed us that we need something called "dental hygiene." [27]

While dental hygiene is important, it isn't as vital to your health as *spinal hygiene*. Poor posture, bad sleeping habits, sitting too much, and all forms of stress act to degenerate your spine just as sugar does your teeth. And just as with dental hygiene, you need to address these deleterious factors on a regular basis if you do not want decay and if you don't want to lose the use of your spine before you hit fifty.[28] Some forms of spinal hygiene include:

- Exercises to strengthen the paravertebral (back) musculature, abdomen, and quadriceps (front of legs), which all become weak or atrophied due to sitting too often.
- Proper stretching of anterior musculature—pectorals (chest) and anterior deltoids (front of shoulders) as well as the calves and hamstrings, all of which poor posture tightens.

To receive the maximum nerve supply you're looking for, you need someone who's aim is spinal correction—not just pain relief. For help in finding the right doctor visit: www.MaximizedLivingMakeover.com.

MaximizedLivingMakeover.com

MAXIMUM MEMORY
Discover how to increase memory by maximizing nerve supply.

Using various methods of evaluation, chiropractors use precise contact points to gently shift segments of the spine and extremities in a very specific direction.

TAKE A STEP FORWARD!

Your spine is your lifeline through which your brain regulates all the activity of your body. All real wellness is ultimately dependent on the spine and nervous system's ability to provide maximum nerve supply.

> Chiropractic adjustments are incredibly safe.

1. Forward Head Posture Syndrome is serious and requires immediate investigation. That's because it can add up to 30 pounds of abnormal leverage on the cervical spine and create the loss of lung capacity, and eventually cardiac, circulatory, and digestive problems. The best way to tell if this is a problem for you is to consult with your nearest Maximized Living Doctor or Mentor.

2. Good posture is not only important to your mother—it's important to your doctor. Don't take posture for granted and don't accept slouching as unavoidable. Not only can poor posture be indicative of problems, it can also cause them.

> Dental hygiene is important, yet it isn't as vital to your health as *spinal hygiene*.

3. A key factor in a healthy spine is the correct "Arc of Life." Losing your Arc of Life causes the most severe obstruction to the central nervous system. If you're not sure if you have the proper Arc of Life, or if you've never had a spinal X-ray, it's important to get one right away from your Maximized Living Doctor or Mentor. The faster you act, the quicker you can begin to remove the interference and allow the body to start healing itself.

4. Because the spine is so important to good health, it makes sense not only to correct any problems, but also to practice good spinal hygiene. Your Maximized Living Doctor or Mentor can evaluate your condition and design a specific program just for you.

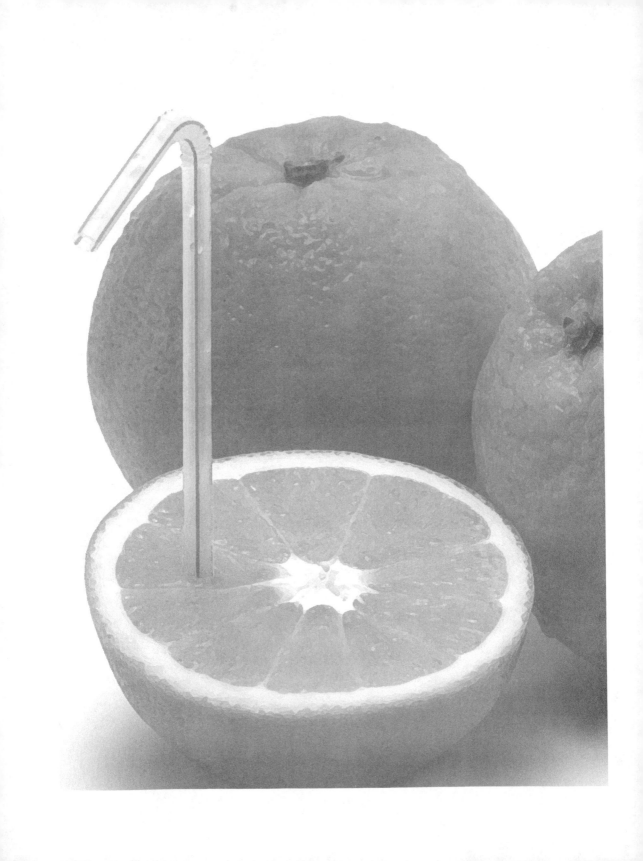

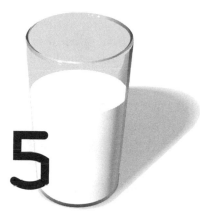

5

ESSENTIAL 3:
Maximize the Quality of Your Nutrients

To efficiently run the numerous and intricate operating systems that comprise your complicated body, each of your forty trillion cells needs fuel. This fuel is in the form of adequate nutrition. Lack of quality food and inadequate levels of certain nutrients will interfere with normal body function and create poor health in any number of areas.

Every cell of your body is made up of what you ingest. The modern diet of convenient, processed, and chemical-laden meals poses a serious threat to healthy cell life. Thus, most people's heart cells are made out of McDonald's French fries and Krispy Kreme donuts.

These cells are floating in body fluids that come from what you drink. For that reason, the quality of the liquids you consume is vital for supporting life. Bathing your organs (*organ*-ized cells) in coffee; cola; impure water; and red, green, and purple drinks also badly interferes with your state of wellness. If fish can't survive in a bowl filled with those beverages, what makes you think *your* cells will?

Maximized Living Makeover .com

MaximizedLivingMakeover.com

YOU ARE WHAT YOU EAT!

Watch this outstanding video to get the inside scoop on the typical American meal and the true definition of "healthy eating." From a pepperoni pizza and a diet cola with ice cream, to a whole wheat turkey sandwich— know what you are eating!

> Each of your forty trillion cells needs fuel. This fuel is in the form of adequate nutrition.

MaximizedLivingMakeover.com

WHY DIET SODAS MAKE YOU FAT

Read a special report on the latest research by Dr. Charles Majors.

Essential 3 is a call to become considerate of your body and conscious of what you are putting into it in order to help create maximized living. This rule is in close relationship to essential 1. Your body is a divine mix of chemical reaction after chemical reaction. When you dump foreign chemicals in the body, the side effects can be explosive.

> SAD REALITY—The U.S. diet is called the Standard American Diet or SAD.

- Sixty-one percent of American adults are overweight.
- One billion people worldwide are overweight, which Congress called "as serious a threat as global warming."[29]
- In the past twenty years, overweight children ages six to eleven have doubled—tripled for adolescents.
- The U.S. will have three new generations of degenerative illness in the near future.
- A twenty-two-pound weight gain (the average middle-age weight gain) increases heart attack risk by 75 percent. A fifteen-pound weight gain doubles your risk of developing type 2 diabetes.

Myth: When you get older, you get fatter...and slower...and dumber.

Truth: This is common in the United States but definitely not normal. You can make changes now to lower these statistics when it comes to you and your family.

Diet or Nutrition?

Most of today's nutrition guidance has been diluted down to the term *diet*. This is due largely to the fact that people have gotten so large. With obesity on the increase, it's no wonder that when you talk about healthy eating, people think of the latest fad diet. The catch-22 is that

> The quality of the liquids you consume is vital for supporting life.

the health and diet industry is, in part, responsible for the current outrageous level of obesity!

In recent years, diet books have ruled the top of the charts, you can sign up for dozens of different online diet programs and join dozens more weight loss clubs. All promise quick, permanent weight loss. Yet obesity has skyrocketed, including going into hyperspace for kids: nine million kids under the age of six are now obese! With all of the promises that guarantee losing weight—someone's lying.

A dramatic shift from home-cooked, natural foods to fast, convenient foods is ultimately responsible for so many people being overweight. On the other hand, diet programs undoubtedly haven't worked and have really just made us fatter. With so many of these programs using refined, prepackaged foods or other unhealthy methods to lose weight, you get thinner, but not healthier. You may lose weight, but if you're also not healthier all that means is you die lighter! That, or you don't keep the weight off anyway. Maximized Living is leading people back toward making better choices about what they put in their mouths and using actual facts about nutritional needs and not fads. As all of the Five Essentials do, eating the Maximized Living way supports and does not interfere with the laws that govern function and healing.

"Max Food"

When you consider only taste or filling yourself up when you eat, you are simply ignoring a major law of life. Equally important is making sure the diet is unique for your needs and that you can actually follow it. We have beginner, intermediate, and elite (advanced healing) level diet plans that hundreds of thousands have been able to apply successfully based on their individual abilities and situations. They are packed with the foods you were intended to eat that we call "Max foods."

Max foods are the foods that grow and exist in nature. They were created with all the necessary materials in just the right amounts and in the perfect balance for proper digestion, distribution, and elimination of nutrients.

MaximizedLivingMakeover.com

MULTIVITAMINS
Are they needed? Watch this special video to cut through the hype and get to the help! What foods will help? What are good pills? Bad pills?

> If a fish can't survive in a bowl filled with coffee; cola; impure water; and red, green, and purple drinks, what makes you think *your* cells can?

The further away the food is from nature, the more toxic and nutrient-deficient it is. The purpose of food is to provide fuel for your cells, not only to satisfy taste. Obtaining pleasure and flavor from food is highly possible and important as long as we don't fail to forget this purpose for food. Unfortunately, we mostly eat foods that have been dramatically altered through commercial farming and food processing. We forget food's purpose in lieu of convenience and getting addicted to the taste of all of those flavorful chemicals.

The body's digestive system is an intricate network of food-assimilating organs whose purpose is to break down and utilize the food you eat. All the organs of this system have unique cells, glands, fluids, and functions that are naturally formulated to play a specific role in the amazing manner in which the very demanding human body absorbs food.

When you take in maximized food or Max foods in their natural state, the digestive system will easily break them down, dispense the nutrients to body cells, and quickly eliminate leftover toxins and by-products. No *dis*-ease is created or developed.

Man-Food

Man-food is food human beings create or alter. It is also food not intended for humans to eat on a regular basis. These processed man-foods break essentials 1 and 3 as you pound your body with chemical poisons. Like medications, these food toxins create imbalance in your internal ecosystem that can only end up eliciting dangerous side effects in your body.

Many types of man-food are recommended by different diets. These fad programs utilize unnatural foods and prepackaged foods containing processed animal products, chemical containing powders and meal replacements, and certain stimulant supplements. They may produce weight loss short term and, in very rare cases, even long term. They don't, however, produce health; you probably won't make it long term.

The further you get from eating the foods specifically created for the body, or the farther these foods are from their natural form, the less efficiently the digestive system can break them down—if it can at all. This poisons the body (breaks essential 1), interferes with function and healing (breaks essential 3), or in other words causes poor health, sickness, and disease.

Foods that cannot pass through the digestive system quickly and cannot be broken down efficiently will linger inside your body. This will block the processing of other nutrients, rob you of energy, contaminate your cells, create excess fat storage, affect your moods, and contribute to every type of symptom and disease known to humanity.

Even if man-foods list vitamins and minerals on the label, few if any are truly usable. Anything that is devoid of nutrition or life is unlikely to be able to *sustain* life. It's too far removed from the purpose it was meant to serve.

The body has multiple protective mechanisms for cleaning out toxins and restoring harmony. This can keep you alive or at least breathing for a time. Unfortunately, man-food will not allow you to breathe too well or for too long.

Important: Don't panic when you see the man-food list! We don't want crash dieting or rebound weight gain from the thought of giving up chocolate. In fact, with the upcoming "vacation rule," you can still eat chocolate.

The Max Diet Plans
Simple, Beginner, Intermediate, and Elite
(the Advanced Healing Diet)

The Simple Max Diet

The Simple Max Diet isn't really even a diet. In fact, we call it an *un*diet. It's particularly effective for children and people who have newer issues with weight and poor health who simply need to clean up their act. The simple plan is especially helpful for people who work in an environment where it is very challenging to make good food choices 100 percent of the time.

The simple diet works like this: Simply eat as often as possible from anything on the Max food list while being aware of the "carbohydrate" issue. There are two simple steps.

Nine million kids under the age of six are now obese! With all of the promises that guarantee losing weight—someone's lying.

"MY DAD'S STORY"

is one of the most poignant testimonials you will ever read about the tragic consequences of not even trying to live a Maximized Life. Read this powerful story by Dr. Ben Lerner.

1. The 80/20 rule—The first, basic step to cooperating nutritionally with Maximized Living is to eat all or the majority (80 percent good, only 20 percent bad is the 80/20 Rule) of your meals off the Max food list.
2. Eat your carbs early; eliminate your carb addiction—Eat carbs in the morning or in the early part of the day.

One of the fiercest enemies to good health and a lean body is unused carbohydrates. If you eat a bowl of pasta and some bread at night, you've just eaten enough carbohydrates to run a marathon. Instead, you go to bed and these unused carbs wreak havoc on your glands. The abundance of sugars they create overwhelm the insulin mechanisms necessary to absorb them, and they end up stored as fat. All this results in you getting up in the morning feeling more tired than you were when you went to bed.

In the morning, it has typically been six to twelve hours since you have fueled up, and you still have an entire day ahead of you. Therefore, energy foods can be used up. Keeping the majority of your carbs in the morning gives you ample time to burn what you've taken in and leaves little left over for storage in the gut or butt.

Vegetables, Proteins, and Fats—
Eat in increasing amounts all day long

Protein—builds and repairs broken-down muscle and tissue. Because the body has been at rest, it doesn't have a significant need for proteins (building and repairing) in the morning. The morning is more of a carbohydrate-dense, good fat meal, whereas the afternoons and evenings should be the protein-dense meals.

Fats—support cell structure and healing. But large amounts of fats with large amounts of carbs make you fat. Because the body has been resting all night and because breakfast is a carb meal, fats should be added to the morning meal but kept to a moderate-to-low level. Good fats are those found in fish, avocado, walnuts, flax, olive oil, wild fish, and organic-grass fed meats. These assist in the function of both the immune and cardiovascular systems. They're also important in protecting joint and brain tissue.

Bad fats, on the other hand, can be a foe of well-being. Bad fats include hydrogenated oils—nut, vegetable, and seed oils—and saturated fats from commercial meats.

Six Rules to Help You Make These Simple Changes

1. **The Addition Rule**

   Rather than making a lifetime commitment to good eating overnight and taking away bad food (that you really like), start by adding good food and you'll make a positive difference. The addition rule states that instead of eliminating the bad, you will add the good. So if you drink diet soda and eat a candy bar for breakfast every morning, you should not stop that behavior and start eating nothing but fruit. If you do, you will only quit the diet—or your brain will explode—whichever comes first.

   What the addition rule has you do is add an apple to your cola and candy bar breakfast. With the addition rule, you do not take away; you *add*. As we stated, most people are overfed but undernourished. By adding healthy foods, you become not only fed but also nourished.

   When you are told to "eliminate" something, it gives you an instant attachment to it and you only want it more. Noticeably, there is no "rule of elimination" anywhere in the undiet.

   Over time, you will react so positively to these additions that you will begin to crave the healthier items as opposed to only the unhealthy ones. Gradually, those nutritional items that were once merely additions could become the entire focus of the meal.

2. **The Replacement Rule**

   The world is full of tempting treats that create a large amount of craving and satisfaction but offer little nutrition. Traditional favorites such as pizza, ice cream, cookies, sodas, sugared cereal, fast food, and other unhealthy choices are literally addictions and create a real dilemma when trying to make proper

> You may lose weight, but if you're also not healthier all that means is you die lighter!

MaximizedLivingMakeover.com

BMI CALCULATOR
and what it means.

decisions. To help avoid caving in to these cravings and addictions, the undiet suggests an effective nutritional theory known as the "replacement rule."

Many of the junk foods listed above, in their original form, contain harmful ingredients that break the laws of life. However, today's modern health food and grocery stores offer a variety of substitutes you can buy or make that are similar in form, satisfaction, and taste to these foods.

Using this rule, you will soon find yourself more and more satisfied with the healthier substitutes to your cravings. Eventually, you may even be able to eliminate these cravings altogether. To help you, here is a handy list of common food cravings and their replacement foods:

> Max Foods are the foods that grow and exist in nature. The further away the food is from nature, the more toxic and nutrient deficient it is.

REPLACEMENT FOODS	
Craving/Addiction	Replacement Food
Pizza: store-bought or homemade	Whole grain pizza with all-natural sauce and low-fat, unrefined cheese
Ice cream	Low-fat, frozen yogurt
Sugary, refined cereal	One of the many health food, whole grain cereals with rice or almond milk
Coffee	Coffee Substitute: herbal tea, heated chocolate or vanilla almond milk
Sugar	Honey, fresh fruit juice, unrefined maple syrup, molasses, brown rice syrup
Rich desserts	Whole grain, nondairy, chemical-free, low-fat, honey or fruit-sweetened treats
Fast-food burger	Lean, homemade all-beef burger lean turkey burger, or veggie burger
Store-bought cheese	Organic or raw cheese

3. Everyone's Favorite Rule: The Vacation Food Rule (You Don't Cave If You Crave)

If eating well creates too much stress, it negates many of the positive benefits. The vacation food rule was created as a way of making the process of change much less stressful and much more fun.

Many people are either on a diet or off a diet. The undiet, however, is not a diet at all. It is a way of eating that is something to work on for the rest of your life. No matter how satisfying your work, you need an occasional break. The vacation food rule puts a food, a meal, or even a whole day of the less-than-ideal food choices into your week. The idea that "if you crave, you cave" is a myth. Rather than calling it "cheating" when you give in to a craving, occasionally eating poorly is actually part of the undiet plan.

While occasionally you will take a spontaneous vacation, the best vacations are planned. Therefore, suppose you are an ice cream lover. Well, if you eat ice cream every day, you are going to get fat. However, if you utilize the vacation food rule, you set a short-term goal for when you *will* eat the ice cream. You may say, "I will eat ice cream only on Wednesdays and Sundays." Then, on Tuesday, when you pass your favorite ice cream parlor or somebody asks if you want to try their cone, you can resist your craving and say, "No thanks, I eat ice cream only on Wednesdays and Sundays."

Some cravings are so great, they are difficult to handle. By setting a short-term goal, you usually can push yourself over the hump and make it another day or two. Another positive side effect of this rule is that often when you isolate only certain days to eat some of your cravings, you will find that you do not feel well after eating them. You may discover that you have a food sensitivity to these vacation foods that you never knew about before when they were mixed in with other meals.

MaximizedLivingMakeover.com

Take a trip down
THE DIGESTIVE
TRACT
to learn how your body processes food.

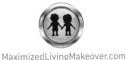

4. **The Food Dress-Up Rule**

Initially, many of the healthier food choices may not seem very appealing. Max foods tend to appear less tasty and fulfilling because of all the additives, sugars, salts, and fats that give less healthy, man-made foods their flavor. The reality is that natural foods do possess good taste, but our taste buds have been dulled due to all the flavorings and spices in man-made food.

In order to make healthy food more palatable to your abused and desensitized taste buds, use the food dress-up rule. For instance, oatmeal is a healthy breakfast choice generally free of all the toxic foodstuffs that dilute and debilitate many other breakfast foods, such as cereals and donuts. The challenge is that oatmeal by itself does not contain much flavor, and preparing it with man-food like sugar will negate some of the positive benefits. Yet simply eating oatmeal and hot water every morning can become a real chore for most people. Even the most avid of oatmeal fans would become tired of just straight oatmeal and honey after a while. To make this nutritious breakfast more appetizing, simply prepare "cool oatmeal."

Cool oatmeal is your standard oatmeal with different *healthy* items added to dress it up. Adding berries, almonds, cinnamon, raw butter, and/or low-fat granola will dress up the oats and make them more attractive.

After a period of using Max foods, eventually the sensation will return to your taste buds, and foods will require less dressing up.

5. **The Stay Full Rule**

Food choices are triggered by something called "hunger." *When hunger signals reach a high enough level, it will be almost impossible to make good decisions.* That is why the stay full rule states that the way to achieve proper nutrition is not to get too hungry.

Consuming regular, healthy meals at appropriate times of the day achieves a proper balance of staying nourished while also staying satisfied. On the other hand, skipping meals and going hungry lead to a practice of becoming "starved" and create the need for eating anything within reach to satisfy the inevitable hunger pangs.

What is most satisfying and often most available are those heavily refined, fast, or fried foods that are full of fat. To avoid consuming such "junk" food, always stay full throughout the day with good food.

6. **The Multiple Feedings Rule**

To achieve the stay full rule, it helps to also follow the multiple feedings rule. This last theory of proper nutrition states that smaller, lighter, healthier meals should be eaten throughout the day to avoid the intense hunger associated with weight loss.

Most folks eat two or three relatively large meals a day. However, the body is better equipped to process small amounts of food every few hours. Large amounts of food cannot be handled well by the body and can cause loss of energy, digestive dysfunction, and fat storage. Going long periods of time between meals also slows down the metabolism, making you even less likely to burn these large amounts of calories. Multiple small- to medium-size feedings take less energy to digest, burn well, and speed up the metabolism. To achieve ultimate results, eat four to six times a day.

Now you have new rules for eating, which you will get to try when you take the thirty-day Intermediate Makeover Challenge in the back of the book. It's time to take a look at the next undiet, the Max Beginner Diet.

The Max Beginner Diet

The first two Max Simple Diet steps—the shift to the Max foods list and the elimination of addiction to carbohydrates, particularly in the afternoons and evenings—will make a major change in your health and body. To begin now making even larger gains in health and leanness, it's time to move from the Max Simple Diet to the Max-3 Diets—beginner, intermediate, and elite (also called the Advanced Healing Diet). After making even the beginner diet changes to the

> Man-food is food human beings create or alter. It is also food not intended for humans to eat on a regular basis.

MaximizedLivingMakeover.com

BOUNCING BACK AFTER PREGNANCY

Do you have to add "baby weight" to the twenty-two-pound average weight gain of middle-age years? Watch Dr. Sheri Lerner and other women who have "bounced back" tell you how you can beat the odds, too!

way a person eats, more than 90 percent of people will get amazing results. Chances are, you'll want to keep going.

Here are the three beginner changes that everyone should make to experience maximized living:

The Three Beginner Changes

There are many nutritional changes you need to make. However, we found that these three beginner changes to your diet are undoubtedly the most effective and critical. The first two changes are very simple to implement because they are horizontal shifts in our eating habits. The third change is trickier, but it can be done over time.

1. If you are eating man-made fats, simply replace them with good, nonman-made fats.
2. If you are eating man-made meats, simply replace them with good, nonman-made fats and meats.

Note: These two changes take very little effort beyond educating yourself about your new food choices to replace the old ones.

3. If you are eating processed grains and refined sugars, remove them from your diet.

This is definitely the most challenging step and should be implemented after making changes in the first two. This change may be the most difficult, but it will yield the greatest transformation in your health.

Set time goals to implement each change. For example, transition to eat all good fats and meats in sixty days and remove all refined and processed sugars in ninety days. Let us explain why implementing these three eating rules in the Max Beginner Diet is so important by looking at each change in detail:

MAX BEGINNER CHANGE #1:
Remove bad fats. Replace with good fats.

Bad fats, such as hydrogenated and partially hydrogenated oils, trans fats, and rancid vegetable oils are linked to cellular congestion leading to cancer, chronic fatigue, and neurotoxic syndrome. Bad fats are also linked to chronic inflammation, which is the key to twenty-first-century medicine. Heart disease, stroke, cancer, diabetes, and other diseases are the leading causes of death in the United States, and inflammation is at the root.

On the flip side, good fats are the most lacking nutrient in the Standard American Diet (SAD), not vitamins and minerals. Good fats are essential to hormone production, cancer prevention, brain development, weight loss, cellular healing, and anti-inflammation.

We know that all the talk about fats in the media has made many Americans believe that all fat is bad. That's just not the case. But some fats are very bad. Your job with the help of the Max Beginner Diet changes is to learn the difference and start using the good fats—in the right way. See if you already know the truth about fats by examining these Max myths vs. truths:

Myth: Fat makes you fat.

Truth: Fat does not make you fat. It's your body's inability to burn it that makes you fat. Fat burning is regulated by a hormone called leptin, which is explained in the Max Advanced Diet.

Myth: Butter is bad.

Truth: Butter contains arachidonic acid, which is important for cellular and brain function. Butter also contains CLA, which aids in fat burning.

> Foods that cannot pass through the digestive system quickly and cannot be broken down efficiently linger inside your body. They block the processing of other nutrients, rob you of energy, contaminate your cells, create excess fat storage, affect your moods, and contribute to disease.

> The first, basic step to cooperating nutritionally with Maximized Living is the 80/20 rule— eat 80 percent of your meals off the Max Food list.

Myth: One bag of French fries now and again will not hurt anyone.

Truth: The half-life of trans fats or hydrogenated fats is 51 days. This means that after 51 days, only half of the negative effects of this man-made fat have been processed. The body needs 51 additional days, or a total of 102 days, to remove the majority of the trans fats and their negative effects, such as decreased nerve transmission, decreased focus and an increase in hyperactivity. Other negative effects include decreased immunity and an increased risk of cancer, diabetes, and heart disease.

As you can see, not all fats are automatically bad for you. In fact, your body needs fats—but it needs the right ones used in only the right ways. Cooking fats changes their molecular structure and must be done at the proper temperatures in order to keep good fats from becoming bad ones.

Tip: Cooking with fats and oils without turning good fats into bad fats

HIGH HEAT: Use only coconut oil, olive oil, grape seed oil, or rice bran oil for frying. The best choice is coconut oil because of its superior flavor when frying food such as chicken. Olive oil, while just as healthy, tends to make food soggy rather than crispy. A word of caution regarding olive oil: It will turn rancid when heated above 120°F. If it smokes, it has already turned rancid.

MEDIUM HEAT: To sauté foods, use sesame oil, rice bran oil, olive oil, grape seed oil, coconut oil, or butter.

BAKING: Butter, coconut oil, sunflower, safflower, or olive oil can be used in baking if the temperature is less than 325°F. In a hotter oven, only use butter, olive oil, or coconut oil. If coating a pan or cookie sheet, use only coconut oil or grape seed oil.

NO-HEAT OILS: Cold-pressed oils such as Body-BioBalance, flax oil, hemp seed oil, sunflower oil, and safflower oil should not be heated but can be added to food after it is cooked.

⚡Note: A NOTE ABOUT HEMP OIL: Hemp oil has nature's ideal four-to-one omega-6 to omega-3 ratio and is recommended to be used two times daily, mixed with food that contains protein. Examples would be to mix the oil in stews and soups (cold), sauces, salad dressings, casseroles, nut butter, and so on.

⚡Note: Refrigerate hemp oil and all cold-pressed oils.

MAX BEGINNER CHANGE #2:
Change the meats that you eat.

Hundreds of studies link commercial meats with cancer and heart disease. When grain is fed to animals that were created to eat grass, it changes the fatty-acid ratios and denatures good fats in the meat, leading to modern-day disease. Add to that the bioaccumulation of commercial pesticides, herbicides, antibiotics, and hormones in meats, and you have a recipe for health disasters. Levels of these toxins are far higher in meat than what you receive from commercial vegetables. This leads to many cancers and chronic illness.

It's also FDA approved for stores to sell animals injected with steroids, antibiotics, and other drugs and even sell cloned meat without any warning on the labels!

Grass-fed and free-range meats offer many fatty acids missing in the Standard American Diet (SAD) such as: arachodonic acid, congegated linoleic acid, and the proper ratio of omega-6 and omega-3 fatty acids.

These organic, grass-fed and free-range meats are hard to find at typical grocery and health food stores. Therefore, they need to be ordered. It's somewhat more expensive so you may not be able to eat them at every meal. But doing something is much better than nothing.

MaximizedLivingMakeover.com

FOOD DRESS-UP RULE
Learn some favorites of Dr. Ben Lerner's and share your own!

MaximizedLivingMakeover.com

LABEL READING
How to spot hydrogenated and partially hydrogenated oils in your foods. When is 0 percent not 0 percent? How can you avoid misleading labeling?

Max Facts: The Science Behind the Meat and Fat

Scientists are now realizing that the ratio of fatty acids like omega-3 and omega-6 is more important than the single fatty acid itself. In grass-fed cows, for instance, the ratio is two to one to four to one of omega-6 to omega-3.[30] In grain-fed cows, this important ratio is twenty to one or higher. Similar effects occur in grain-fed chickens and their eggs. In this case, more is definitely not better. The danger of fat ratios that far exceed what occurs in nature is contributing to a myriad of health problems in both children and adults.

In children, these unnatural fat ratios are causing slower brain development and an all-too-common set of complicating symptoms we refer to as ADHD[31]. But they are no less damaging to adults. Excessive omega-3 to omega-6 ratios contribute to a host of ailments including heart disease, cancer, hormonal issues, skin conditions, and type 2 diabetes, just to name a few.

Myth: Saturated Fat in meat causes heart disease and cancer.

Truth: It's not the meat; it is what man has done to it. Saturated fat contained in grass-fed meat is critical for brain and cell function. Studies even indicate that the saturated fat in grass-fed meat prevents heart disease.[32]

MAX BEGINNER CHANGE #3:
Remove *all* processed grains and refined sugars from your diet.

Sugar is an antinutrient offering insignificant amounts of vitamins and minerals and robbing your body of precious nutrient stores. This inevitably leads to diseases of the new millennium such as chronic fatigue, ADD, ADHD, heart disease, diabetes, and cancers.

Remember that refined sugars unnaturally spike and elevate insulin and leptin. Prolonged spiking and elevation of insulin and leptin lead to insulin and leptin resistance.

Insulin and leptin resistance cause diabetes and weight-loss resistance or the inability to burn fat for energy, respectively. High-glycemic or refined sugars cause elevated glucose, which elevates insulin leading to premature aging and degenerative diseases such as type 2 diabetes, heart disease (inflammation of the arteries), and cancer.

Removing processed grains and refined sugars seems tough, because they are everywhere. Yes, this includes white rice, white pasta, and white bread. These are processed grains that turn into "sugar" and raise glucose and insulin the same as sucrose, fructose, or any other "-ose."

To identify acceptable grains, the words *whole, stone-ground,* or *sprouted* must be before the word *wheat* or other grain's name. For example, if it doesn't say the words whole wheat, it is processed. Wheat flour is not a whole grain and is thus disease-causing to your body.

One-third of sugar consumption comes from soft drinks, while two-thirds of our sugar intake comes from hidden sources including: lunch meats, pizza, sauces, breads, soups, crackers, fruit drinks, canned foods, yogurt, ketchup, mayonnaise, and other common foods.

Truth: Removing all refined sugar is by far the hardest of the three beginner changes, but it is equally as important as the others, partly because most Americans are addicted to sugary foods. To our bodies, sugar is a drug. If there is any lingering doubt of this fact, just talk to someone who gave up sugar and experienced classic detox symptoms like headaches, shakes, gastrointestinal trouble, fatiguem and mood swings. These symptoms alone should serve as a warning about how dangerous sugar is to the body.

Truth: With sugar removed from a child's diet, the child will experience less sickness, fewer behavior issues, better sleep, and better grades. Experience has shown that it takes about one week for cravings for sugar and breads to cease. Any indulgence in sugar during this time, no matter how small, will trigger cravings. Therefore, I tend to adopt an "all-or-nothing" approach to sugar.

> Keeping the majority of your carbs in the morning gives you ample time to burn what you've taken in and leaves little left over for storage in the gut or butt.

YOU NEED FAT!

An in-depth report from
Dr. Ben Lerner

Tip: Removing all sugar at once is easier than a little at a time because you lose cravings in approximately five days as the result of insulin and leptin receptor regeneration.

Truth: Refined sugar lowers the immune system.

Now let's see if you know the truth about refined sugar:

Myth: I eat very little sugar, and I am still overweight.

Truth: Americans consume an average of 120 pounds sugar per year, per person, compared to 5 pounds per year, per *family* in the early 1900s. These sugars are hidden in virtually every boxed food, cereal, and cracker. Fruit juices that are labeled "100-percent juice" typically contain more sugar than a can of soda.

Tip: Look at the sugar content on labels. Anything with *-ose* at the end is sugar.

Tip: TIPS: Avoid corn syrup, fructose, sucrose, malt, barley malt, maltodextrin, dextrose, sweetened brown rice syrup, rice syrup, and sugar cane. (The herb Stevia and Xylitol are acceptable sweeteners.)

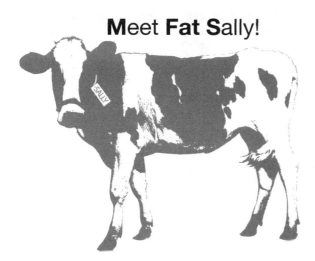

Meet **Fat Sally!**

TO REMEMBER THE THREE CHANGES:

1. Meet—Change to grass-fed meat!

2. Fat—Change from bad fats to good fats!

3. Sally—Change to whole grains and remove all processed grains and sugars!

In order to change your bad eating habits to good ones, it's important to know what foods are the right ones to choose, especially if you are a beginner. We have put together several lists to help you make good food choices that will set you firmly on the path to maximized living!

Max foods List
Maximize your food choices using the Max foods Beginner Diet Quick List

Max Proteins Choices
Choose raw (not roasted nuts and not pasteurized or homogenized cheese) grass-fed, free-range, cage-free, and no-hormone-added sources whenever possible. Avoid farm-raised and Atlantic fish.

> Good fats found in fish, avocado, walnuts, flax, olive oil, wild fish, and organic grass-fed meats assist in the function of both the immune and cardiovascular systems.

GRASS FED AND
FREE RANGE
What you need to know.

HERE ARE SOME MAX PROTEIN CHOICES	
Cold-water fish (salmon, sardines, Mahi-Mahi, mackerel, etc.)	Game birds (pheasant, duck, goose, grouse)
Eggs	Ricotta cheese
Cottage cheese	Beef
Raw cheeses	Lamb
Chicken and turkey	
Vitol egg protein	Venison
Whey protein: must be raw	

Max Good Fats Choices

As with proteins, choose raw (not roasted nuts and not pasteurized or homogenized cheese), cold-pressed, grass-fed, free-range, cage-free, and no-hormone-added sources whenever possible. (If you want peanut butter, look for the Valencia brand.)

Grass-fed meat	Avocado
Coconut or Flakes	Butter
Cod liver oil	Grape Seed Oil Vegenaise (a mayonnaise replacement)
Hemp oil (three-to-one ratio)	Raw cheeses
Olive oil, olives	Full-fat coconut milk, oil, and spread
Flaxseed oil	Full-fat raw milk
Grape seed oil	Full-fat plain yogurt
Almond butter	Eggs
Lydia's Organics Grain-Free Crackers	Cashew butter
Canned sardines in oil or water	Raw nuts and seeds: Almonds, cashews, flax, hemp, pecans, pine nuts, macadamia, sesame, sunflower, walnuts, etc.

⚡**Note:** Absolutely avoid hydrogenated and partially hydrogenated oils such as cottonseed oil, soybean oil, and vegetable oils; trans fats such as margarine and synthetic butters; rancid vegetable oils such as corn oil, canola oil, or those labeled simply vegetable oil located in practically every bread, cracker, cookie, and boxed food!

Max High-Fiber Carbohydrate (Vegetable) Choices

Choose organic when possible. Remember, the best carbohydrate choices are vegetables due to high-fiber content and low-glycemic action. This means there is little to no glucose or insulin rise when consumed.

Arugula	Collard greens	Mustard greens
Asparagus	Coriander	Onions
Bamboo shoots	Cucumber	Parsley
Bean sprouts	Dandelion greens	Radishes
Beet greens	Eggplant	Radicchio
Bell peppers (red, yellow, green)	Endive	Snap beans
Broadbeans	Fennel	Snow peas
Broccoli	Ginger root	Shallots
Brussel sprouts	Green beans	Spinach
Cabbage	Hearts of palm	Spaghetti squash
Cassava	Jicama (raw)	Summer squash
Cauliflower	Jalapeno peppers	Swiss chard
Celery	Kale	Tomatoes
Chayote fruit	Kohlrabi	Turnip greens
Chicory	Lettuce	Watercress
Chives	Mushrooms	

Starchy Carbohydrate Choices

Choose organic when possible. If weight loss is a concern, eat starchy carbohydrates in moderation. These carbohydrates have a moderate glycemic action. This means they do cause a small to moderate glucose or insulin

Start your undiet by adding good food, and you'll make a positive difference.

MaximizedLivingMakeover.com

IS FOOD MARKETED AS "ORGANIC" REALLY ORGANIC?

Learn what to look for and who to trust.

rise when consumed. The foods italicized are grains. In the beginner plan these grains must be whole. The grains with an asterisk (*) are Max grains—the only grains permissible on the Max Intermediate Diet.

Squash (acorn, butternut, winter)	Black beans	Split peas
Artichokes	Chick peas (garbanzo)	White Beans
Millet*	Rye	Semolina (whole grain, dry)
Leeks	Cowpeas	Yellow beans
Lima beans	French beans	Tapioca
Barley	Steel-cut oats	Whole-grain breads
Okra	Great northern beans	Bulgar (tabouli)
Pumpkin	Kidney beans	AkMak crackers
Buckwheat groats (kasha)	Amaranth*	Ezekiel bread (sprouted)
Sweet potato or yam	Lentils	Wasa crackers
Turnip	Mung beans	Non-GMO corn*
Brown rice*	Spelt	Corn
Legumes	Navy beans	Whole-grain cooked cereals
Adzuki beans	Pinto beans	Whole grains
Wild rice*	Quinoa*	Whole-grain tortillas

Max Fruit Choices

Choose organic when possible. If weight loss is a concern, eat fruit in extreme moderation.

MAX FRUITS CHOICES			
Berries (blackberries, blueberries, boysenberries, elderberries, gooseberries, loganberries, raspberries, strawberries)			
Avocados	Lemons	Limes	Granny Smith apples

MODERATION FRUITS			
Cherries	Oranges	Pitted prunes	Passion fruit
Pears	Peaches	Apples	Persimmons
Fresh apricots	Plums	Nectarines	Pomegranates
Melons	Grapefruit	Tangerines	Kiwi

SPARING FRUITS		
Eat sparingly after a workout with some protein. Avoid if weight loss is a concern.		
Banana	Grapes	Mango
Pineapple	Watermelon	Papaya

Max Eating Tip: Eat More Vegetables

Note: Potatoes are not vegetables. They are tubers that raise glucose and insulin, especially if white.

Tip: If you cook vegetables, lightly steam them. Raw is best.

Tip: Some people will do better with more protein and fewer vegetables, and others will do better with more vegetables and less protein, depending on their metabolic or genetic type (for example, an Eskimo vs. a Peruvian Indian).

Tip: Organic is best. If not organic, wash them with distilled vinegar or solution available in health food stores. Use bags to squeeze air out of the vegetables before storing.

Tip: Always eat some protein with vegetables (for example, an egg or piece of chicken, turkey, or fish)

Tip: Add in a good "greens" powder product that you put in your water if you do not get six to nine servings of vegetables per day. This is a whole-food vegetable supplement designed for this purpose.

The vacation food rule puts a food, a meal, or even a whole day of the less-than-ideal food choices into your week.

MaximizedLivingMakeover.com

ADD AND ADHD.
If your child has difficulty focusing, this special report from Dr. Charles Majors contains urgent information you need.

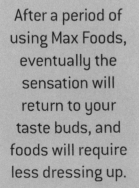

After a period of using Max Foods, eventually the sensation will return to your taste buds, and foods will require less dressing up.

Tip: Prepare weekly menus with lots of variety.

Make a menu for each week; Sundays are the best time for many people. If you work, make meals ahead of time. Make enough for leftovers. Wash and bag veggies on Sunday for one week. They will stay fresh if you use vacuum bags with zip locks.

To add variety to your diet, find ten recipes that you like. If you rotate between only two or three meals, boredom will threaten your success.

Note: Listen to your body. Your cravings and energy levels will tell you when you need to adjust or modify your personal plan. However, during the first two weeks while insulin levels are adjusting, you will need to eat more meals a day to feel better.

The Max Beginner Diet is for everyone, and these three steps move you toward maximized living. By choosing to make these three changes, you are choosing a lifestyle of energy, health, strength and longevity. If you desire to go to the next level in maximizing your health, explore the power in the Max Intermediate Diet and the Max Elite (Advanced Healing) Diet.

The Max Intermediate Diet

The Max Intermediate Diet is a powerful diet researched and formulated to maximize your body's full potential for health, energy, recovery, and brain power. This is accomplished by continuing the Max Beginner Diet and now refining it to eat only Max grains (one meal a day) and Max fruits. These minor alterations provide maximum benefits to metabolism, glucose and hormone regulation, as well as your body's immune response to foreign protein, such as gluten and cellular nutrition.

The Max Intermediate Diet follows the same food list and principles as the Max Beginner Diet with the following limitations:

The Max Intermediate Diet was created through grain research that shows genetically altered grains are so altered that many individuals have intolerances or allergic reactions to the grain proteins. Historically, when a culture consumes 50 to 60 percent of its calories from grain, degenerative diseases rise proportionally. The Max Intermediate Diet limits your grain intake to one meal a day and specifies healthy grains that are less altered by man.

These grains include: Wild rice, brown rice, quinoa, millet, amaranth, and non-GMO corn. Why these grains? They are mostly ancient grains that have less genetic alteration, more nutrients, more protein, less intolerance (gluten-free), and lower glycemic action.

From the Max food Beginner Diet List Choose only Max fruits. These are best ingested after a workout and with protein such as a grass-fed, nonpasteurized, or nonhomogenized raw whey protein.

For the Max Intermediate Diet, it's highly recommended that you take the plunge and go organic. Why? Because organic fruits, vegetables, nuts, and seeds contain higher nutrient levels and avoid the use of cancer-causing chemicals.

Tip: Blending vegetables increases nutrient uptake and therefore increased energy, clarity, and metabolism, supporting weight loss.

Truth: Removing grains that contain gluten (found in wheat and wheat products) significantly decreases the symptoms of ADD/ADHD, asthma, allergies, autism, ciliac, and other digestive disorders.

For many, the Max Intermediate Diet is the ultimate diet to maximize your life. However, there are some individuals who need the Max Elite (Advanced Healing) Diet to optimize body function.

The Max Elite (Advanced Healing) Diet

Some individuals require a more advanced diet to restore health and healing to their body. I call this diet the

> The stay full rule states that the way to achieve proper nutrition is not to get too hungry.

MaximizedLivingMakeover.com

SUGAR-PRODUCING FOODS AND ALKALINE VS. ACIDIC FOODS

Test what you know! View a chart to see the best foods for your body!

> To avoid consuming "junk" food, always stay full throughout the day with good food.

Max Elite Diet otherwise known as the Advanced Healing Diet. Five factors will determine if this diet is right for you. Many individuals needing this diet are already in a state of disease, such as ADD, autism, cancer, chronic fatigue, fibromyalgia, diabetes, or heart disease, to name a few. However, this diet is also used by others on a short-term basis for detoxification and weight loss and on a permanent basis for those who are genetically suited for this diet.

Why is this diet so powerful and what makes it work?

The Max Elite Diet works utilizing two principles: increasing good fats and removing sugar and everything that turns to sugar (grains). These principles allow this diet to do three things for your body that no other diet can do.

Three Functions of the Max Elite Diet

Following this diet accomplishes three objectives: healing and powering up the fifty to one hundred trillion cells that make up your entire body and thus controlling inflammation, assisting in the removal of toxins, and regulating hormone function.

1. Inflammation—The Max Elite Diet controls inflammation throughout your body. This type of inflammation affects every organ, tissue, artery, blood vessel, hormone, and cell, and therefore determines your state of health. Studies indicate that inflammation is the root cause of the number-one killers in America and the majority of the degenerative disease we are facing today. For example, the true cause of heart disease is not cholesterol but an inflammatory condition of the arterial wall. Removing grains from your diet controls inflammation by eliminating a sugar called amylose. Amylose is present in all grains except corn and causes an inflammatory reaction, particularly in individuals suffering with inflammatory conditions (heart disease, arthritis, chronic fatigue, fibromyalgia, and irritable bowel syndrome, to name a few).

   As scientists and doctors look for the next miracle cure, they should look no further than controlling this type of inflammation. However, the cure will not lie in the form of a pill but will come from these dietary changes and detoxification.

2. Detoxification—The Max Elite Diet achieves detoxification because it heals the cell membrane. True detoxification must occur at the cellular level. Nutrients must move in and toxins must come out in order for a cell to be clean and healthy. The cell membrane is the gatekeeper that allows this to occur. The Standard American Diet (SAD) and our toxic environment cause the cell membrane to be inflamed. When the cell membrane becomes inflamed, the above process is hindered. The cell becomes toxic. To restore and heal a toxic cell, you must remove sugar and everything that turns to sugar. This regulates insulin and an enzyme involved in controlling cellular inflammation called PLA2. Regulating insulin and PLA2 controls cellular inflammation. This is the key to true detoxification.

3. Hormone regulation—Controlling inflammation (cytokines and PLA2) and removing toxins allow hormone receptors on the cell and hypothalamus, the control center of your brain, to heal and regenerate. Regenerating the receptors allows disregulated hormones to balance and normalize. Most doctors treat hormone disregulation by trying to balance individual hormones. This Max Elite (Advanced Healing) Diet, along with our Maximized Living detoxification protocols, treats upstream to get to the cause all hormone disregulation.

If you have any or all of these five factors, the Max Elite (Advanced Healing) Diet is a must for You:

1. High triglycerides/cholesterol—If you are a sugar burner and not a fat burner, your body will not store or burn fat normally, therefore elevating triglycerides. (100 to 135 is normal. A number greater than 135 means cholesterol levels are elevated.)

> Smaller, lighter, healthier meals should be eaten throughout the day to avoid the intense hunger associated with weight loss.

2. High blood pressure—Inflammation of the large arteries leads to high blood pressure. Inflammation is controlled by the healing diet.

3. Elevated glucose/insulin/leptin—Once the insulin receptors are burned out, a fasting glucose, insulin, or leptin test will be elevated. Removing all sugar is the only way to heal the insulin receptors.

4. Neurotoxicity—A Maximized Living doctor can determine this with a neurotoxic history and visual contrast sensitivity (VCS) test.

Tip: Difficulty losing weight is a neurotoxic clue. Toxins attach themselves to fat cells and continually elevate the hormone leptin. Leptin is the hormone that tells your brain to burn fat for energy. Toxins can burn out leptin receptors in the brain, leading to leptin resistance. As a result, you gain weight that does not respond to diet and exercise.

5. Protein/fat genetic type—Some individuals genetically do better without consuming grains. Others excel on high-fat and/or high-protein diets. This can only be determined by how you feel and how your body responds (weight change, energy, brain clarity, and so on) on a particular diet.

Tip: A family history of diabetes or obesity is a genetic clue that the Max Elite (Advanced Healing) Diet is the perfect diet for you.

The Five Basics of the Elite (Advanced Healing) Diet

The basic idea: We must eliminate *all sugars* and *everything that turns to sugar* to heal the hormone (leptin and insulin) receptors.

Your body needs fats, but it needs the right ones used in the right ways.

- No sugars—this includes all sugar forms!
- No grains—not even whole, healthy grains! (Read the ingredients.)
- Fats—two to three weeks after beginning program. (This is the typical time needed to become a fat burner.)
- No fruits—berries only in moderation and best consumed within one hour of exercise with protein such as a grass-fed whey protein.
- Protein intake—on average should be 15 to 25 grams per meal.

*On average, 20 grams per meal for men or 15 grams per meal for women. Larger men and those performing resistance exercises can consume between 25 and 30 grams per meal.

How do you know how many grams makes a meal? Here are a few pointers:
- An egg typically contains 7 grams of protein.
- A piece of meat the size of a deck of cards typically contains 15 grams of protein.

Two Stop Checks

If you are not losing weight or any one of the five factors is not improving, check the following:
- Check your protein intake. Are you eating too much protein?
- Consider toxicity as a major problem.

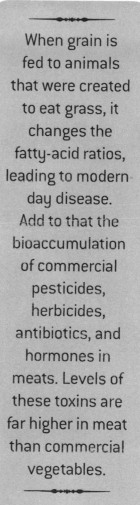

When grain is fed to animals that were created to eat grass, it changes the fatty-acid ratios, leading to modern-day disease. Add to that the bioaccumulation of commercial pesticides, herbicides, antibiotics, and hormones in meats. Levels of these toxins are far higher in meat than commercial vegetables.

To remember the five basics of the Max Elite (Advanced Healing) Diet, find out…

How Sally Got So Fat!

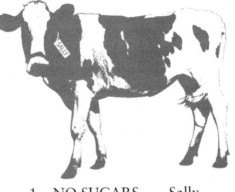

1. NO SUGARS — Sally
2. NO GRAINS — Got
3. FATS   — Fat
4. NO FRUITS   — From
5. PROTEIN   — Pumpernickel

Cows like Sally become fat when force-fed grain, making the meat fat and tasty, yet, deadly.

Here is the Max Elite (Advanced Healing) Diet Food Choice Quick List:

Protein Choices

Choose raw (not roasted nuts and not pasteurized or homogenized cheese) grass-fed, free-range, cage-free, and no-hormone-added sources whenever possible. Avoid farm-raised and Atlantic fish.

> Grass-fed and free-range meats offer many fatty acids missing in the Standard American Diet.

Cold-water fish (salmon, sardines, Mahi-Mahi, mackerel, etc.)	Game birds (pheasant, duck, goose, grouse)	Whey protein (raw, grass-fed) (brand names PaleoMeal™ or Whey Cool™)
Eggs	Chicken and turkey	Beef
Cottage cheese	Vitol egg protein	Lamb
Raw cheeses	Ricotta Cheese	Venison

Tip: Pacific and Alaskan salmon are the best choices. Plus, the smaller the fish, the cleaner the fish.

Fat Choices

Choose raw (not roasted nuts and not pasteurized or homogenized cheese), cold-pressed, grass-fed, free-range, cage-free, and no-hormone-added sources whenever possible. (If you want peanut butter, try the Valencia brand.)

Grass-fed meat	Olive oil, olives	Almond butter
Coconut or flakes	Flaxseed oil	Butter
Eggs	Grape seed oil	Avocado
Cashew butter	Grape Seed Oil Vegenaise	Raw cheeses
Lydia's Organics Grain-Free Crackers	Coconut milk, oil, and spread	Full-fat raw milk
Canned sardines in oil or water	Cod liver oil	Full-fat plain yogurt
Hemp oil (three-to-one ratio)		
Raw nuts and seeds (almonds, cashews, flax, hemp, pecans, pine nuts, macadamia, sesame, sunflower, walnuts, etc.)		

> To identify acceptable grains, the words *whole*, *stone-ground*, or *sprouted* must be before the word *wheat* or other grain's name.

Note: As in all of the Max diets, absolutely avoid hydrogenated and partially hydrogenated oils such as cottonseed oil, soybean oil, and vegetable oils; trans fats such as margarine and synthetic butters; rancid vegetable oils such as corn oil, canola oil, or those labeled simply vegetable oil, located in practically every bread, cracker, cookie, and boxed food.

Tip: Cod liver oil is best ingested in the winter due to the naturally high vitamin D content.

High-Fiber Carbohydrate (Vegetable) Choices

Choose organic when possible. Remember, the best carbohydrate choices are the vegetables below, due to their high-fiber content and low-glycemic action. Eat as much as you desire or until full.

Arugula	Collard greens	Mushrooms
Asparagus	Coriander	Mustard greens
Bamboo shoots	Cucumber	Onions
Bean sprouts	Dandelion greens	Parsley
Beet greens	Eggplant	Radishes
Bell peppers (red, yellow, green)	Endive	Radicchio
Broadbeans	Fennel	Snap beans
Broccoli	Garlic	Snow peas
Brussel Sprouts	Ginger root	Shallots
Cabbage	Green beans	Spinach
Cassava	Hearts of palm	Spaghetti squash
Cauliflower	Jicama (raw)	Summer squash
Celery	Jalapeno peppers	Swiss chard
Chayote fruit	Kale	Turnip greens
Chicory	Kohlrabi	Watercress
Chives	Lettuce	

Carbohydrate Choices in Moderation

These carbohydrates can be consumed in small amounts and not on a daily basis.

Artichokes	Black beans	Lentils
Leeks	Adzuki beans	Mung beans
Okra	Chick peas (garbanzo)	Yellow beans
Pumpkin	French beans	Pinto beans
Tomatoes	Great northern beans	Split peas
Turnip	Navy beans	White beans
Legumes	Kidney beans	Lima beans
Squash (acorn, butternut, winter)		

One-third of sugar consumption comes from soft drinks, while two-thirds of our sugar intake comes from hidden sources.

Max Fruit Choices in Moderation Only

Choose organic when possible. If weight loss is a concern, eat fruit in extreme moderation.

Berries (blackberries, blueberries, boysenberries, elderberries, gooseberries, loganberries, raspberries, strawberries)			
Avocados	Lemons	Limes	Granny Smith apples

Tip: Max fruits are best consumed within one hour of exercise with protein such as a grass-fed, whey protein.

Low Fiber Carbohydrates to *Eliminate*

These carbohydrates are moderate to high glycemic, with little fiber to regulate the glycemic action. They turn to sugar very quickly, so do not eat them.

Barley	Tapioca	Wasa crackers
Brown rice	Whole-grain breads	Whole-grain tortillas
Buckwheat groats (kasha)	Whole-grain cooked cereals	Sweet potato or yam
Bulgar (tabouli)	Quinoa	Sprouted grains
Millet	Spelt	Amaranth
Rye	Whole grains	Wild rice
Semolina (whole grain, dry)	AkMak crackers	Ezekiel bread
Steel-cut oats		

Note: If you are not concerned with weight loss and are on this diet because of neurotoxicity, non-GMO corn is permissible because it does not contain amylose and therefore will not cause an inflammatory response unlike the whole grains listed above.

Tip: Eliminating sugar is critical! Refined sugar lowers the immune system.

> With sugar removed from a child's diet, the child will experience less sickness, fewer behavior issues, better sleep, and better grades.

MaximizedLivingMakeover.com

Share your favorite
MAX DIET RECIPE
and win free resources!

Sugar promotes yeast growth.

One can of soda has nine to eleven teaspoons of sugar. Avoid corn syrup, fructose, honey, sucrose, maltodextrin, dextrose, molasses, rice milk, almond milk, fruit juice, sweetened brown rice syrup, maple syrup, dates, sugar cane, corn, beet, and lactose. (The herb Stevia and Xylitol are acceptable sweeteners. However, even Stevia can stimulate carbohydrate and sugar addiction cravings.)

Look at sugar content on labels. Anything with *-ose* at the end is sugar!

For the Max Elite Diet, avoid carbs or sugars from vegetables that are not grown above ground. They will alter insulin levels.

Tip: No more grains!
Stop eating grains until normal glucose and normal weight are reached as prescribed in the Max Elite Diet Plan. It will take several days to lower insulin levels. In the meantime, high insulin levels will cause symptoms such as dizziness, confusion, headaches, and a general ill feeling.

Eating every two hours can help minimize unpleasant symptoms during this transition.

Tip: Eat frequently!
Eating four to six meals a day is better for weight loss, even after your system adjusts.

Eating more frequently has shown to normalize blood sugar levels.

Truth: Your cells can only use two things for energy—fat and sugar. Most Americans are stuck in sugar burning mode and therefore are plagued with uncontrollable cravings.

Truth: Regulating the hormone leptin allows your brain to burn fat for energy and therefore provides freedom from uncontrollable cravings.

Removing all
sugar at
once is easier
than a little
at a time.

⚡Truth: Leptin is regulated when you eliminate sugar and everything that turns to sugar (Max Elite Diet).

⚡Truth: Ninety-five percent of leptin disregulation occurs as a result of toxicity. Therefore, many individuals will not lose weight until true detoxification occurs.

⚡Truth: The Max Elite (Advanced Healing) Diet is a must for any toxic condition and is the diet of choice for everyone using the Maximized Living Customized Nutrition Program detoxification protocols. For a doctor who can help you tailor a CNP, go to www.MaximizedLivingMakeover.com. For sample meal plans and menus, turn to part three.

Weight-Loss Resistance

Why We Got So Big and Have Trouble Getting Back to Small

If the current trends continue, 100 percent of the U.S. population will be obese by the year 2230.[33] Excess weight is an established risk factor for high blood pressure, type 2 diabetes (adult onset), high-blood cholesterol level, coronary heart disease, and gallbladder disease.

The question is, "Are we really eating that much more than we were a decade ago?"

The biological fact is we are not. Our calorie consumption doesn't match up with this enormous, exponential rise in obesity. It's really the onslaught of refined, toxic foods; an excess of sugar and sugar-based preservatives in our diet; an enormously sedentary lifestyle; and, equally important, our stressed and rushed culture, which has created the "weighty" predicament we're currently in.

These issues listed have created an assortment of "metabolic damage" factors that have created additional weight gain. If you've tried to lose weight and struggled, you probably suffer from weight-loss resistance. These metabolic factors make it extremely difficult if not impossible to lose fat.

In 90 percent of people, just doing the Simple or Beginner Max Diet will resolve their weight issues and even solve the

> Historically, when a culture consumes 50 to 60 percent of its calories from grain, degenerative diseases rise proportionately.

ACID REFLUX

Does it keep you up at night? Read this special report from Dr. Ben Lerner.

> The true cause of heart disease is not cholesterol but an inflammatory condition of the arterial wall.

weight loss resistance issues. But there is a segment of the population that has damaged its metabolism to the point of being severely weight loss resistant. These people must heal these areas before their body will really be able to burn fat and hold onto or build lean tissue.

Why Is Weight Loss So Important?

The scientific community was recently shocked when the *New England Journal of Medicine* released several studies showing that being moderately overweight, even if you have no symptoms of poor health, increases your mortality rate (chance of dying early) by 30 percent.

In order for your body to lose weight, the hormones insulin and leptin must be doing their work. Insulin is in place to control sugar and fat storage levels in the body, while leptin's job is the burning of fat. If these hormones and the mechanisms that are there to utilize them aren't working, you will be unable to lose weight. Plus, you will be extremely prone to packing it on.

Let us look further at the two reasons these hormones begin to fail in your body:

1. Too many sugars and grains (essential 3)—When you eat sugar, processed grains, and even healthy grains, they're converted to sugar. In order to absorb this sugar, insulin is secreted by the cells of the pancreas. If insulin is always elevated, it blocks fat burning, lowers serotonin (which results in feelings of depression), causes internal fat storage around the abdomen and causes inflammation within the body.

2. Toxins (essential 1)—Toxicity is perhaps the greatest problem in the fight to lose weight. When toxins enter your body, they have an affinity for fat cells, due to the fact that they are fat soluble. When the toxins attach to the outer cell membrane that is made of a lipid bilayer (two layers of fat), it causes the cells to continually release leptin.

When leptin is elevated too often, just like insulin in type 2 diabetes, the receptors burn out and the message is not heard. If leptin is out of balance, despite your best efforts, you will not lose weight. The toxins also cause the release of chemicals called cytokines that damage leptin receptors in the brain (hypothalamus). Once the receptors to leptin have been damaged, weight-loss resistance is only the first of many problems.

Your body also makes an extremely important hormone called MSH (melanocyte stimulating hormone). MSH is produced in the hypothalamus by leptin, and it controls nerve, hormone, cytokine functions, skin and mucous membrane defenses, as well as controlling the production of endorphins and melatonin. If your brain cannot hear leptin (leptin resistance), you will eventually become MSH deficient.

What does all this mean? It means that every immune and hormone response in your body will be altered. Practically speaking, you feel horrible and cannot figure out why. You find yourself on medications, chasing symptoms on a never-ending downward spiral.

In many of the Maximized Living Health Centers, a patient history and a blood test are used for measuring leptin to determine what diet is best. By visiting one of these clinics or one that does similar work or by taking the challenge at the end of this book with a qualified leader, you can discover programs and treatments designed to scientifically and effectively rebalance your hormones and get you healthy and at your ideal weight, even if nothing has ever worked for you before!

> The cure for inflammation will not lie in the form of a pill but will come from dietary changes and detoxification.

Weight Loss and the Other Four Essentials

Toxicity is huge, but it works in tandem with *all* of the Five Essentials. We will go into essentials 4 and 5 later, but just look at the effects of stress! Weight gain or loss has as much to do with essentials 1, 2, 4, and 5 as it does with essential 3—food.

Important Stress Effects On Your Physique (Essential 5):

1. Stress raises cortisol, the catabolic hormone that causes you to put on fat, lose muscle, resist insulin, increase appetite, and crave sugar.

MaximizedLivingMakeover.com

HEALING DIET VS.
ATKINS DIET

Dr. Ben Lerner helps you understand the vital differences between Maximized Living and diet fads in this video.

2. Chronic stress lowers serotonin and makes you hypo-glycemic—both of which cause you to crave sugar.
3. Chronic stress affects your body's ability to build muscle. Lean muscle is your "metabolic girdle," which is the key factor for metabolism.
4. Stress depletes B-vitamins so that you can't make the neurotransmitters needed to help you go to sleep and stay asleep.
5. Less sleep elevates cortisol, produces less of the anti-aging hormone melatonin, and gives your body less blood sugar control.

MAX Truth:

1. People who sleep two to four hours a night are 73 percent more likely to be obese.
2. Those who get five hours of sleep are 50 percent more likely to be obese.
3. Those who sleep six hours are 23 percent more likely to be obese.
4. Those who get ten or more hours are 11 percent less likely to be obese.[34]

It's incredible how the effects of stress will sabotage any chance you have at looking and feeling good. Rushing, caffeine, sugar, and continuous emotional turmoil all play a role in causing too much tension and lack of sleep. All of these make it challenging, if not impossible, to lose weight and look good!

The Role of Vitamins, Minerals, and Herbs

Your health coach and wellness doctor may prescribe supplements for boosting immunity and giving you nutrients necessary for repair and recovery. These vitamins, minerals, and herbs can be of great assistance, particularly in the case of toxicity, weakness, damage, or breakdown from unknown, long-term nutritional deficiencies or poor body function.

It's necessary to seek the counsel of a well-informed health professional who can assess your needs and lead you in the right direction. Otherwise, you can overdo certain supplements and are likely to waste a bunch of time and money.

True detoxification must occur at the cellular level. Nutrients must move in and toxins must come out in order for a cell to be clean and healthy.

Remember, essential 3 is "maximize *quality* nutrition." Using discount and drugstore supplements is almost worthless, as they are going to come out of you looking almost exactly the way they looked on the way in. In fact, you might as well throw cheap, nonprofessionally recommended supplements right into the toilet and cut out the middle man.

Wellness professionals typically have quality supplements available. They may cost slightly more than they do at the discount mega store, but nutrients are not a good place to be frugal.

⚡Tip: Just taking an assortment of supplements will rarely ensure you get the ones your body needs. Additionally, it can be very harmful as you overdo some and underdo others.

The Basics

Everyone needs a basic amount of vitamins, minerals, and enzymes found in a good multivitamin. Additionally, few people get enough green foods, clean-usable protein, or omega-3 fats. It stands to reason that everyone's basic supplementation schedule should consist of:

A Multivitiamin/Multimineral Supplement

Think of a high-quality, multivitamin/mineral and antioxidant formula as your proactive health insurance.

Greens Powder or Capsules

You need to eat five or more servings of colorful, organic vegetables every day. The more the better, and quality greens can ensure that you are getting what you need. You will get a synergistic blend of colorful vegetables with no allergenic grains.

Organic Grass-Fed Whey Supplement

Protein provides the building blocks for hormones and neurotransmitters. It is essential that you get an optimal amount of clean, lean protein at each meal. Cool-processed, grass-fed whey is a fantastic source of protein. It is very

Are we really eating that much more than we were a decade ago? The biological fact is we are not. Our calorie consumption doesn't match up with this enormous, exponential rise in obesity.

MaximizedLivingMakeover.com

Find the closest
MAXIMIZED LIVING
HEALTH CENTER
near you!

bioavailable, raises the master antioxidant glutathione and it also helps chelate (bind and pull out) heavy metals.

Omega-3 Supplementation

If you're eating a standard commercial diet that consists of very little grass-fed meat, omega-3 eggs, walnuts, avocado, or fish, then you need to supplement the missing omega-3s in your diet.

It's now common to overdo omega-3 supplementation and end up creating the opposite problem. Therefore, ideally, you should get the majority of these fats from foods recommended in the Max food list of good fats.

Advanced

There are five key factors to consider when it comes to supplementation:

1. Am I taking a *sufficient* amount of nutrients that I need to supplement (vitamins, minerals, amino acids, and fatty acids) in order to be well and not develop disease?
2. Is there something in particular that my body is *deficient* in that I need to take more of in order to be well and not develop disease?
3. Is my body even capable of normal *absorption* of the nutrients I'm taking?
4. Are the supplements I'm using *capable of being absorbed*?
5. Am I possibly *causing harm* to myself due to the amounts, types, or brand of supplements I'm using?

To truly determine the answers to these advanced questions, five-factors testing is needed. This avoids guessing—not getting enough or getting too much of certain nutrients—and stops you from wasting money on what you don't need. You'll also discover you can't take cheap supplements and change a test. There are few legitimate ways to test nutrient deficiency. None are simply done in a doctor's office or health food store. One test that is available is called an Organic Acids Test. This is done by sending a urine sample to a CLIA certified medical lab that specializes in this area.

> Being moderately overweight, even if you have no symptoms of poor health, increases your chance of dying early by 30 percent.

Test-Worthy Areas That We Evaluate through Organic Acid Testing in Our Maximized Living Clinics

With the advantage of testing, you can find out if you are deficient in certain key areas. You may be taking supplements. Testing shows if you are getting a sufficient amount. Insufficiency can be due to a number of factors that are discovered in the tests—the need for more, the need for more quality, and/or an issue with your ability to absorb nutrients altogether.

The following areas and nutrients are key factors studied in the tests and should be addressed in any supplementation program:

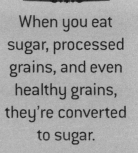

When you eat sugar, processed grains, and even healthy grains, they're converted to sugar.

B Vitamins
- Your body needs them to make energy.
- They are required in detoxification.
- They are needed to make neurotransmitters.
- Deficiencies could cause or exacerbate certain neurological conditions.
- They are necessary for optimal digestive function.

Just rebuilding B vitamin status can improve energy, lower homocysteine, help with depression and improve mood!

Cellular Energy

This area looks at whether your body can create energy efficiently, if you can burn fat easily and if you are building up lactate, which could result in muscle soreness and fatigue. Blocks here could result in poor fat burning, general overall fatigue, muscle aches, and poor exercise recovery. Nutrients that are important here include CoQ_{10}, carnitine, lipoic acid and B vitamins. This category can help improve your overall energy, reduce muscle soreness, and enhance exercise recovery, as well as help you become a better fat burner!

Neural Function

This category relates to neurotransmitters, the chemicals your nervous system uses to function and communicate with your body. Abnormalities in this area can relate to

MaXimized Living
MAKEOVER

SLOWING THE AGING PROCESS
A closer look at lipid peroxides.

symptoms of mental, emotional, and behavioral problems, including PMS, insomnia, anxiety, depression, food cravings, and uncontrollable appetite. Imbalances can be due to stress, poor diet, poor digestion, or nutrient deficiencies. An example of poor neural function: A forty-year-old man complaining of hunger that is "out of control." Favorite expression: "I am starving out of my mind."

Lipid Peroxides

Are you aging faster than you should? Oxidative Stress is one of the things that ages us. It isn't something you can see on a traditional lab test. How much antioxidant protection you need will depend on a variety of factors, including your environment, your stress level, and your diet. Lowering oxidative stress may lower disease risk and slow the aging process.

Your Total Toxic Burden

Have you looked into the Toxic Top Ten? Toxicity can affect endocrine function, especially thyroid function and the ratio of bad proliferative estrogens (E16) to the good estrogens (E2). Toxicity can create weight loss resistance by slowing down metabolism and inhibiting fat burning. Toxicity can increase your risk of cancer, heart disease and neurological disorders.

Dysbiosis

Abnormal overgrowth of unfavorable microflora in the small and large intestines:
- Can cause poor nutrient absorption
- Can cause weight gain and inability to lose weight despite very low-calorie diets, as gut bacteria consume extra calories and store them as fat
- Can cause gas, bloating, diarrhea and constipation

Causes
- Low levels of stomach HCI
- Chronic use of antacids
- Repeated use of antibiotics
- NSAIDS

> Toxicity is perhaps the greatest problem in the fight to lose weight.

- Stress
- Food allergies and sensitivities
- Nutrient deficiencies
- Alcohol abuse
- Immune deficiencies

Fatty Acid Balance

Do you balance your omega-3 fats with omega-6 fats? Low omega-3s are associated with mood disorders. Omega-3s reduce inflammation, help with bone remodeling, benefit your skin, support a healthy mood, and lower triglycerides and cholesterol. Balance is the key! Too much omega-3 fat is as damaging as too little. High omega-3 fats decrease immune function and can increase lipid peroxidation. ENSURE that you are balancing your EPA, DHA and GLA.

Essential 3: The Bottom Line

Congratulations! You have now learned what it takes to rid your body of toxins, feel better, and prevent disease—thanks in large part to essential 3: maximize quality nutrients. You know what foods are Max foods and which ones to eat for the various levels of Max diets. Whether you are following the Simple, Beginner, Intermediate, or Elite Max diets, we promise that you will look and feel better within just a few days of sticking to any one of our undiets! Plus, you will be well down the road to maximized living. You have also taken a crash course in supplementation and discovered how testing might help you get your body in balance.

After we take a look at all the Five Essentials and how they work together, you will have the opportunity to take a thirty-day challenge best suited to fit your health needs and put one of the Max diets to work for you. In the meantime, you have already learned how to minimize toxins (essential 1), maximize nerve supply (essential 2), and maximize quality nutrients (essential 3). Let's take a look in the next two chapters at how the last two essentials work together for you.

> Rushing, caffeine, sugar, continuous emotional turmoil, too much tension, and lack of sleep make it challenging, if not impossible, to lose weight and look good!

MaximizedLivingMakeover.com

FISH OIL
Is your fish oil supplement helping you or hurting you? What you must learn to make sure you're taking a beneficial fish oil supplement.

It's necessary to seek the counsel of a well-informed health professional who can assess your needs and lead you in the right direction.

TAKE A STEP FORWARD!

You are what you eat—literally. That's why it's important to give your body the foods it was designed to eat, the nutrients it was designed to use—at the right times of the day, and in the right amounts.

1. There's a reason they call it "morbid obesity." Every pound counts. That's why it's so important to understand your BMI (Body Mass Index) and act appropriately. If you haven't taken the online BMI test, you should do so right away at www.MaximizedLivingMakeover.com. Be sure to watch the video that explains what the results mean.

2. Diets don't work; in fact, diets often don't even help. Most people who lose weight on a diet end up putting it back on—and a few pounds more. And staples of dieting like diet soda actually create increased cravings and make it harder to lose weight. To lose weight, don't rely on a fad that tries to trick your body, instead fuel your body the way it was designed to be fueled and not only will the pounds come off, you will be healthier and happier as a result. Focus your mind instead on an "Un-Diet" that will lead to lasting, lifelong health.

3. Introduce Max Foods into your diet to start. These are the foods that grow and exist in nature and have all the necessary materials for proper digestion, distribution, and elimination of nutrients. The farther away a food is from nature, the more toxic and nutrient-deficient it is. The website will help you find the foods you need.

4. Eating the Maximized Living way is a journey that starts right where you are.

    - Seek to make 80 percent of your foods Max Foods.
    - When you eat carbs, eat them early in the day.
    - Don't eliminate bad foods, gradually replace them with Max Foods.

- It's OK to take food vacations and occasionally enjoy those favorite foods—even if they aren't Max Foods.
- Help your Max Foods taste even better by dressing them up.
- Eat frequent, smaller meals.

5. The MAX Elite Diet can control inflammation, and aid both detoxification and hormone regulation. Find these foods at www.MaximizedLivingMakeover.com

6. Vitamins, minerals, and herbs are important—so don't economize on them. Quality supplements administered according to your unique needs can boost your immunity and provide the nutrients necessary for repair and recovery. Your Maximized Living Doctor or Mentor not only has high-quality supplements, they can help you determine the exact nutrients you need.

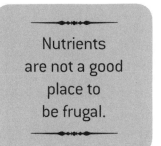

Nutrients are not a good place to be frugal.

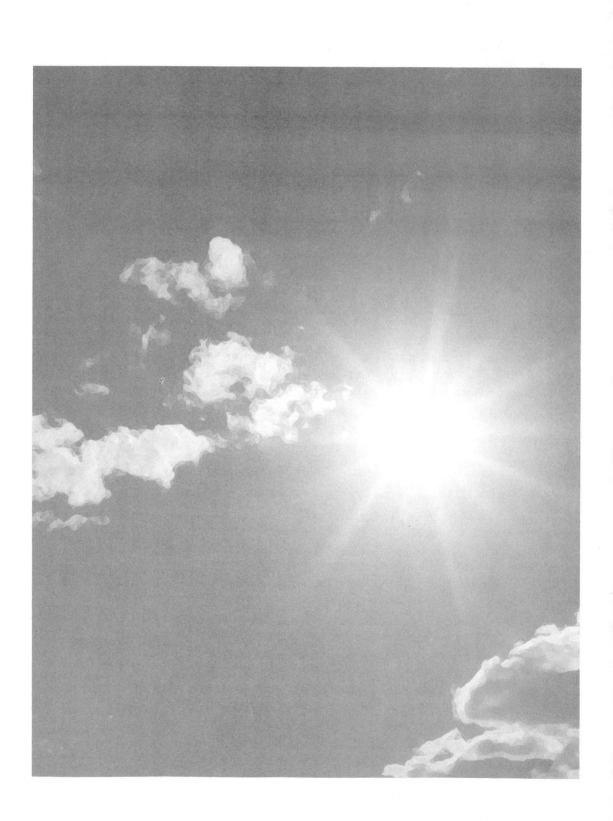

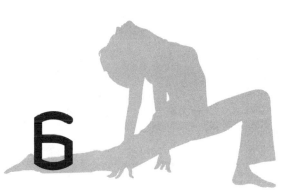

6

ESSENTIAL 4:
Maximize Oxygen and Lean Muscle Tissue

Maximized Living Makeover .com

MaximizedLivingMakeover.com

THE
EXERCISE
PILL

The benefits of exercise are amazing! If a pill created all of these benefits, everyone would want to take it. Watch an in-depth report by Dr. Ben Lerner on all the benefits you experience from exercise.

Although we placed a lot of emphasis in the last chapter on nutrients and supplements, the most important element you need to take for surviving at your max isn't a protein or sugar. It isn't even a carbohydrate or fat. The most important element you need to survive at your max, in fact, to survive at all, is oxygen. You can last quite awhile without burgers or donuts, but you won't make it more than a few minutes without oxygen.

If a cell's environment contains lowered levels of oxygen, it will accumulate toxins, develop disease, and eventually cause early cell death. Your body needs proper amounts of oxygen in every cell to keep them happy and healthy, and there's a simple way to develop the best intake, usage, and storage of oxygen—get up and get moving! That's right. When your body moves, it creates the need in your cells for additional oxygen. And you can take in that oxygen by more movement—also known as *exercise*.

In addition to optimizing oxygen levels, exercise produces muscle. One way to measure health is by how much lean muscle tissue you have compared to fat tissue.

> The most important element you need to survive at your max, in fact, to survive at all, is oxygen.

There's a simple way to develop the best intake, usage, and storage of oxygen—get up and get moving!

Using this measurement, the more muscle you have and the less fat you have, the healthier you are. Many conditions, symptoms, and diseases are set in motion by a body with a low-muscle to high-fat ratio.

Therefore, the benefits of exercise are high and wide. Exercise has even been found to be a viable and at least equally effective alternative to traditional medical treatment of depression.[35] Like all of the other essentials, exercise improves function. There are so many benefits of exercise that it would be impossible to list them all, but here are just a few of the things exercise does for you:

- Improves heart function
- Lowers blood pressure
- Reduces body fat
- Elevates bone mass
- Prevents brain deterioration
- Improves learning
- Slows and even reverses effects of aging
- Decreases total and LDL cholesterol ("bad cholesterol")
- Raises HDL cholesterol ("good cholesterol")
- Raises energy level
- Enhances and balances hormone production
- Aids sleep
- Increases stress tolerance
- Eliminates toxins
- Reduces depression
- Controls or prevents diabetes (blood sugar issues)
- Decreases the risk of injury to the muscles, joints, and spine
- Protects against falls—the number-one cause of death in the elderly
- Speeds up metabolism

In fact, research shows that brisk, moderate physical activity provides up to 50 percent reduction in your chance of forming Parkinson's and many forms of cancers and causes improved function in all metabolic activities.

Falling is the number-one cause of death in the elderly. Resistance training with dumbbells or free-form machines is the best way to develop accessory muscles necessary for balance.

Every vital system in your body that keeps you alive—your heart, lungs, spinal cord, muscles, and arteries—requires that you move on a consistent basis. These systems need exercise to function properly and, in some cases, even function at *all*.

It's actually even better to be overweight but in good shape than it is to be thin but never exercise. A study in 1999 of 25,000 men showed that overweight men who were fit were half as likely to die younger than men who were thin but unfit.

"It's pretty clear that if you follow a healthy diet, don't smoke, but are unfit you are still at high risk of disease and early death," said Steve Blair, author of the study and director of the Cooper Institute in Dallas.[36]

While other research shows that exercise does not completely negate all the dangers of obesity, Blair's study does reveal how important it really is to follow essential 4: maximize oxygen and lean muscle.

Exercise Excuses

Despite the fact that most of us know the benefits of exercise, 87 percent of Americans don't do it on a regular basis—or at all. The top excuses are: "I hate it," "It hurts," "I'm injured," "It's boring," "I don't have the place," or "I don't have the money." The biggest excuse, however, is "I don't have the time."

The right method of exercise beats all the excuses. It actually takes very, very little time to exercise if you do it right and—as with everything else we are teaching—you get the maximum benefit. If you are one of those who already exercise and think you don't need this chapter, think again. It's important for you to keep reading. You may find that you are actually wasting time, as well as not achieving the max out of the effort you are putting in to your exercise routine. Here's what we mean:

> One way to measure health is by how much lean muscle tissue you have compared to fat tissue.

MaximizedLivingMakeover.com

WHAT'S YOUR
BIGGEST EXERCISE
CHALLENGE?
See how others have
overcome it!

Optimum Oxygen Levels

You stay alive by taking oxygen in through the lungs. Once the lungs have the oxygen, the heart and blood vessels pump it out to the rest of the organs. The word *aerobic* means "exercise with air." During aerobic, or what is also called cardiovascular exercise because of its benefit to the heart-lung system, the body needs more oxygen than during inactivity. It also needs it faster than usual. As a result, you maximize the efficiency of the lungs, heart, and blood vessels to take in, deliver, absorb, and store oxygen. In essence, you become a highly efficient, oxygen-acquiring and utilizing machine. Cardio-type movements are those that get your heart rate up and get you breathing—taking in air—more deeply.

Choking Yourself to Death?

When you fail to acquire optimum oxygen levels in the body, you interfere with the body's ability to meet basic oxygen demands. Instead of being a lean, mean, oxygen-efficient machine, your system begins to struggle with its ability to take in, store, carry, and absorb its most important nutrient. This means having higher levels of carbon-monoxide waste in the body; fewer functional blood vessels; and a smaller, weaker heart that beats harder and faster because it is pumping less blood per beat.

As a result of less aerobic activity, the body, which needs oxygen to survive, is less oxygenated; in other words, it is literally *choking to death*.

Signs of Poor Oxygen Acquisition (Choking to Death)

Do you recognize any of these symptoms?

- Fatigue
- Injury
- Memory loss
- Joint and muscle pain
- Infection
- Sleep disorder
- Low blood sugar
- Depression

Many conditions, symptoms, and diseases are set in motion by a body with a low-muscle to high-fat ratio.

- Problems absorbing fat
- Decreased libido
- More difficult menstrual symptoms

As you can see, many of the common symptoms and diseases people suffer from are due to a lack of movement and insufficient oxygen. The risk is that people seek doctors to diagnose these symptoms as a "disease" and prescribe drugs. In reality, you don't have a disease, but your body is in a state of *dis*-ease from a need to recognize some or all of the essentials, including exercise.

> It's actually even better to be overweight but in good shape than it is to be thin but never exercise.

Exercise and the Other Essentials

It is important to recognize that all of the essentials for Maximized Living go hand in hand. In the case of exercise and its benefits, essential 2: maximize nerve supply, plays an integral and preliminary role in the amazing benefits of exercise. Without appropriate nerve supply, the organs affected by exercise will not respond appropriately and optimally. Nerve supply is completely reliant on the alignment and posture of the spine.

If your spine is poorly placed and positioned (vertebral subluxation), then exercise can speed up bone and soft tissue deterioration, cause damage to the vertebrae and nerves, make you more susceptible to joint or muscle injury, and make you more vulnerable to serious spinal cord trauma following a fall or collision.

Anyone beginning or maintaining an active exercise program should be evaluated first by a chiropractor for spine and joint dysfunction.

SURGE Training:
Maximum Exercise for Maximized Living
(Get bikini- and Speedo-ready in just 12 minutes a week!)

How to Overcome the Number-One Exercise Excuse through the Science of "New Aerobics"

For kids like me who grew up in the 1970s, exercise was what your parents did when they just had to lose

OXYGEN
ACQUISITION

Do you have signs of poor oxygen acquisition? Take the survey. Compare your results to others.

> During aerobic, or what is also called cardiovascular exercise because of its benefit to the heart-lung system, you become a highly efficient, oxygen-acquiring and utilizing machine.

weight. The only people who actually exercised regularly as far as we knew were Arnold Schwarzenegger and Lou "the Incredible Hulk" Ferrigno. (Yes, kids, the governor of California and the neighbor on *King of Queens* both used to be bodybuilders.)

Now we realize that being fit is a necessity to be healthy, prevent and overcome disease, and protect our spine and joints. Yet exercise remains for most people more of an annual event than a three-times-a-week one. Again, the mega-excuse for why people don't exercise is that they don't have the time.

The good news is that there is now a method of exercise you can do in only twelve minutes per week without leaving your home or office. It's called SURGE training, and it's the most contemporary thinking on aerobics. Consider it the "new aerobics."

To understand the power of the SURGE, you first have to abandon much of what you've been taught about exercise. Most of us have learned that what is important is what happens to you *during* exercise. In reality, what's more important is what happens *after* you exercise. It's how your body responds that has the greatest impact on your physique and the many layers of your health.

The aerobic craze started back in the 1980s with then-fitness guru Richard Simmons, Jane Fonda, and a whole lot of colorful spandex. Unfortunately, even today people equate exercise with that type of program or fitness video. As a result, exercise has come to mean long periods of time on a treadmill or other piece of cardio equipment. And the longer, the better, right? Thus, the "no-time" excuse. This type of cardiovascular exercise is also known as "low-intensity, long-duration" activity, and to be quite frank, it is an old, outdated, "classic" exercise concept. We'll explain why in just a minute.

Your Delicate Hormonal Balance

Don't you hate the people who can eat whatever they want and never exercise, yet stay skinny or even "ripped"? That's because they have healthy levels of certain hormones acting in their favor. When someone was overweight and used to blame their "glands," we used to say, "Sure, your salivary glands." Now, however, we know that certain hormone deficiencies *do* play a major role in how you look and feel. Classic cardio actually *lowers* these hormones.

The first is human growth hormone (HGH). This is a popular hormone taken illegally by athletes to lower body fat and build muscle and performance. Your body makes this naturally, and you want it to be present in your system in optimal amounts. HGH is essential for fat mobilization. It signals fat-burning enzymes, aids muscle mass development, and is raised the most during sleep. HGH is released in the body in direct proportion to exercise intensity.

Taking this hormone unnaturally, as many athletes and those looking for a fountain of youth do, can be dangerous or ineffective. Boosting your body's own release of this hormone, however, is safe and effective.

The body's desire and ability to release HGH and testosterone, another muscle-building, fat-burning hormone, increase during resistance exercise and high-intensity exercise. Therefore, walking but never adding weight training or resistance machines does not allow for the raising of these hormones. In fact, low-intensity exercise lowers them!

The other set of hormones to consider are "stress hormones." These have the opposite effect of HGH and testosterone. When they are present, you lose muscle and put on fat. Long, stressful bouts of exercise increase stress hormone production—and that's bad.

That's why classic aerobic exercise does harm, as well as good. If you consider the following pros and cons of classic aerobic exercise as most of us know it, I'm sure you'll see why it's time to throw out the spandex, the cassettes, the Richard Simmons videos, and Jane Fonda.

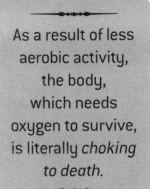

As a result of less aerobic activity, the body, which needs oxygen to survive, is literally *choking to death.*

Effects of Long-Duration, Low-Intensity Classic Aerobic Exercise

Pros of Long-Duration, Low-Intensity "Classic" Aerobics *During* Exercise
- Lowers resting heart rate and increases stroke volume

HGH

Pitchers take it, sluggers rely on it! Should you be injecting it? Read all the latest research by Dr. Charles Majors.

> Many of the common symptoms and diseases people suffer from are due to a lack of movement and insufficient oxygen.

- Lowers blood pressure
- Keeps brain young by increasing circulation to the brain
- Aids detoxification by stimulating the lymphatic system

Cons That Occur *After* Exercise
- Raises stress hormones: The stress hormone cortisol stimulates appetite, is catabolic (breaks down muscle), increases fat storing, and slows down or inhibits exercise recovery.
- Decreases testosterone and human growth hormone (HGH)—both necessary for building muscle and burning fat
- Decreases immune function

Therefore, while there are a few benefits to classic aerobic activity, overall what you're left in is a broken-down, fat-storing, muscle-wasting state. And after all that work too! This is why we hear our patients and readers complaining all the time that they've been exercising and exercising, yet can't seem to lose any weight.

Research done on both elite and novice athletes shows that the benefits of low-intensity, long-duration activity are far outweighed by the benefits of high-intensity, short-duration activity. That's what we have labeled SURGE training.

The Powerful Effects of High-Intensity, Short-Duration Exercise
- It's been shown that HGH release in the body is proportional to the intensity of the exercise.
- Fat is burned in greater quantities after high-intensity exercise due to the release of HGH.
- The beta-endorphin levels increase (giving people positive changes in mood following exercise) during short-duration, high-intensity exercise. (In other words, it's better than an antidepressant!)
- It increases growth of all muscle fibers and slows down the muscle wasting typically attributed to aging.

- Plus, you get all of the health benefits, the "pros," that come with long-duration, "classic" aerobic activity too!

With high-intensity, short-duration exercise, your body responds by increasing the hormones and physiology you need to burn fat and produce muscle. As a result, you not only build muscle and burn fat *during* exercise, but also your body responds by maintaining these benefits for hours *after* you exercise.

Plus, the more muscle you have, the greater the tendency there is to produce more muscle. It's muscle—not age, gender, or genetics—that is the greatest determining factor for good metabolism and future muscle development.

Plus, *plus*, if you can combine this with an aerobic effect, you'll get the benefits of classic aerobics without the negative side effects. That's why we call SURGE training the "new aerobics."

With all these pluses, we bet you'd like to get down to business. If SURGE training is so great for your body and takes so little time, exactly how do you do it?

SURGE Training: High-Intensity, Short-Duration Exercise—the "New Aerobics"

SURGE training consists of intermittent bursts, or surges, of energy. It's similar to the concept of interval training, only done within a more limited time frame and with a strong focus on the importance of the recovery time.

The idea of the SURGE is to safely shock your body into responding physiologically so that you're left afterward in a more ideal metabolic state for getting toned and in better condition. After a maximum energy output, or SURGE, the body must respond. After a SURGE, it responds or adapts by altering hormones and physiology so that your body is burning fat and building muscle during and after the exercise activity.

Anyone can do SURGE training, and it's safe. We can say this because it is built around the fact that your maximum output is what is right for you. You can go at

> Most of us have learned that what is important is what happens to you *during* exercise. In reality, what's more important is what happens *after* you exercise.

EXERCISE VS. PILLS

Which is the better antidepressant? The statistics will surprise you! Read what Dr. Greg Loman has compiled to keep your mind healthy.

Human growth hormone is taken illegally by athletes to lower body fat and build muscle and performance. Your body makes HGH naturally, and you want it to be present in your system in optimal amounts.

---

a maximum without using heavy weights or overstraining your joints or muscles. It's a superior workout for anyone from a beginner trying to drop pounds to the Olympian or professional athlete trying to compete at the highest level. Here's how you get started.

Maximum Heart-Rate Calculation

Before you begin exercising, it's vital to find your training heart rate through the following calculation:

1. Subtract the number of your age from the number 220. The difference equals your maximum heart rate per minute. (For example, 220–40 years old = 180 beats per minute maximum heart rate)

2. During and just after the SURGE training process, your pulse should be 75 to 85 percent of your maximum heart rate. This is your training heart rate. (From the example above, 75 percent of 180 = 135 beats per minute, while 85 percent = 153 beats per minute.)

3. Add 10 to your training heart rate if you're an experienced athlete. As an elite athlete, you can go at or even above your maximum.

4. Subtract 10 if you're a beginner or experiencing or recovering from health problems. You'll need to start a little slower than your maximum.

Note: Stop the workout if you're not an elite athlete and your heart rate reaches 100 percent or more of your training heart rate, and always consult a physician before beginning any new exercise program.

Exercising in "SURGES"

The reason SURGE training is so exciting and can be done by anyone is that in a SURGE set, you exercise as hard as you can (do a maximal output) for a minimum of just ten to fifteen seconds and a maximum of sixty seconds (elite athletes only). Sixty seconds! Anyone can exercise for sixty seconds, right? And it's pretty easy to give up sixty seconds for exercise too. Plus, after just a few of these SURGE sets, your body will begin achieving all of the benefits listed.

After a SURGE set, the secret is to recover just long enough to allow your heart rate to approximate normal or resting heart rate—then you SURGE again. Recovery time is usually equal to the effort time. After the SURGE, you'll find out why even this short amount of exercise is still "aerobics." Aerobic means exercise with air, and you'll definitely be breathing more heavily and seeing your cardiovascular system getting a workout if you are surging at your maximum output.

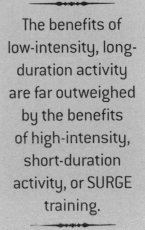

The benefits of low-intensity, long-duration activity are far outweighed by the benefits of high-intensity, short-duration activity, or SURGE training.

Basic SURGE Program

Here are ten basic examples of SURGE training methods. (You will exercise using the SURGE method when you take the challenges at the back of this book.) Remember that the forms of exercise may not look any different than the ones you may have tried in the past. It's the *way* you exercise—in short bursts called surges—that makes SURGE training work.

1. Using a stepper alone or while curling or lifting weights from your hips to your shoulders, up over your head and then lowering the weights to your hips again
2. Stepping up and down on a step, without weights or while using weights as described in #1
3. Riding a bicycle or stationary bike
4. Running outside or on a treadmill without weights
5. Running in place in a pool, with or without water weights
6. Walking
7. Stepping up and down in place on the floor as fast as you can, with or without weights
8. Swimming laps in a pool
9. Rollerblading
10. Using an aerobic machine like a rower or elliptical machine

MaximizedLivingMakeover.com

Check out the interactive
MAXIMUM HEART
RATE CALCULATOR

With high-intensity, short-duration exercise, your body responds by increasing the hormones and physiology you need to burn fat *during* exercise, but also your body responds by maintaining these benefits for hours *after* you exercise.

The SURGE

Here is an example of a SURGE:

1. Twenty seconds of full-on exercise (Get your heart rate quickly up to the Training Zone.)
2. Twenty seconds of rest (Use this full recovery time to get heart rate back to the bottom of the Training Zone or below.)
3. Repeat this cycle three times—twenty seconds on, followed by twenty seconds off after the first two surges.
4. Follow the third surge with two minutes off, as recovery time is important to achieve the full SURGE effect.
5. Now repeat this entire cycle three times, which means you are performing three minutes of total exercise three times. That's approximately nine minutes total elapsed time.
6. Repeat these SURGE workouts four times a week, and watch the results! That equals just twelve total minutes of full-on exercise, with thirty-six minutes total elapsed time!

With SURGE training, who can use "no time" as an excuse for not getting healthy and in the best shape of your life? Let's put it this way: what works better for your busy schedule—three minutes a day of exercise or twenty-four hours a day of being dead?

SURGE training is the most flexible, adaptable, and easy-to-fit-in exercise model with maximum benefits for your life! And it works for everyone. More advanced athletes can work this into their weekly trainings and/or increase the number of surges per session to radically improve their performance times. And surge times can be increased until experienced athletes are doing sixty-second surges.

CAUTION: A sixty-second surge should only be attempted by elite athletes. Once you've gone past a peak output and begin to level off, you lose some of the SURGE benefit and are now doing an "interval." Intervals are effective, but as your body loses the "shock" value, they are not as effective in producing the hormonal response.

Lean Muscles Building:
Adding Optimum Lean Muscle to Your
SURGE Training

One of the many preposterous aspects of the weight-loss phenomenon is the idea of dieting without exercise. You've seen the ads. Lounging around the house eating Big Macs yet losing pounds and inches sounds wonderful, but the reality is that losing weight without increasing muscle means only that you'll fit in a smaller coffin. There are a whole lot of skinny people in the cancer and heart disease wards.

You do not have a weight problem only when you weigh too much; you also have a weight problem when you have too much body fat compared to the amount of lean muscle tissue. Too high of a fat-to-muscle ratio and your body is a prime target to develop disease, even if you don't look overweight.

One of the many aims of exercise is to increase the amount of real muscle and decrease the amount of loosely packed muscle, or what we call *fat*. High body fat-to-muscle ratios negatively affect organ function, hormone balances, immune control, brain activity, and blood chemistry, and that makes you more sensitive to potentially hazardous food elements such as sugar and cholesterol. In our clinics, we test the ratio between fat mass and fat-free mass as a key indicator to longevity and well-being.

Typically, people will walk or jog and call that their exercise plan. The problem is that those exercises don't do a whole lot to build lean muscle. In fact, they can cause muscle breakdown. For muscles to become stronger, leaner, and better developed, you have to apply resistance to them. While many people put resistance only against their gluteus muscles (the ones they sit on), to create muscles you must apply some sort of force.

Your muscles were created for digging, climbing, and wrestling, not simply cracking open a soda. If you do not regularly put your muscles under some strain, you interfere with what it takes to have vital health. When you apply pressure over time, lean-muscle-mass-to-body-

It's muscle—not age, gender, or genetics that is the greatest determining factor for good metabolism and future muscle development.

Combine SURGE with an aerobic and you'll get the benefits of classic aerobics without the negative side effects.

MaximizedLivingMakeover.com

PERFECT POSTURE
Watch Dr. Charles Majors show you how to set up the right way for exercise.

SURGE is a superior workout for anyone from a beginner trying to drop pounds to the Olympian or professional athlete trying to compete at the highest level.

fat ratios go up. This creates a stronger, shapelier body—which isn't bad either!

Some of the Many Benefits of Building Muscle Mass
- Improves glucose tolerance and increases insulin sensitivity, giving you a better chance in the fight against diabetes
- Preserves physical balance, flexibility, and function
- Protects against falls
- Creates a bigger metabolic afterburn from aerobic exercise, allowing you to burn calories and fat long after you're done working out.

The amount of lean body mass you have is the most important factor—above age, sex, or genetics—in determining your metabolism.

Understanding the Language of Resistance Movement through Weight Training
The world of resistance weight training brings with it its own unique and special vocabulary. Such terms need to be defined before a proper understanding of the weight resistance program can occur. They include the following:

Repetitions (or reps)
In the vernacular of weight training, a repetition is defined as how many times you *do* the specified exercise. If you lift a weight twelve times, that is twelve repetitions, or "reps."

Sets
A set is how many separate times you perform the repetitions of the exercise. For instance, three sets of twelve repetitions is performing twelve repetitions, three separate times, or thirty-six total movements.

Failure
Doing an exercise until "failure" means performing a set until your muscles literally cannot perform even one more rep.

Warm-up

Stretching that should occur before every cardiovascular workout or weight resistance training session.

Intensity

Intensity means an exercise is more challenging. However, be forewarned, that doesn't mean you have to use heavy weights or perform workouts that are unsafe or more painful. While adding heavier weights to your sets will increase the intensity of your training, too much weight can also cause pain and injury. The safest way to increase the intensity of a workout is to shorten the time between sets or shorten the time between each exercise. In this way, intensity not only makes your workouts more effective, it makes them more time efficient as well.

Bottom Line for Maximized Living
The more intense your workouts are, the faster you will see results!

Posture + Stretching + Counting + Breathing = Safe and Effective Exercise!

How to Stand: Perfect Posture = Perfect Technique

Exercise and stretching, as well as all movement in life, need to be performed in a state of as close to perfect posture as possible. The body is a high-tech design, utilizing the laws of science, mathematics, and physics in order to best deal with gravity. When you maintain perfect posture, the muscles, joints, and bones are at their strongest and most stable. This will allow them to be able to withstand large or repetitive forces without suffering injury.

Perfect Posture—A Refresher

Remember from essential 2 what perfect posture looks like? Here's a quick refresher:

- The head is up and back so the ears line up over the shoulders, and the arc (lordosis or reversed "C" curve) in the neck is maintained.
- Shoulders are rolled back in the joints.

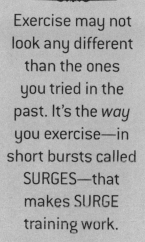

Exercise may not look any different than the ones you tried in the past. It's the *way* you exercise—in short bursts called SURGES—that makes SURGE training work.

What works better for your busy schedule—three minutes a day of exercise or twenty-four hours a day of being dead?

MaximizedLivingMakeover.com

Learn *many* exercises and
SURGE TRAINING!

- The upper back should be flat, not arched or humped.
- The belly button is out and hips back so you have an arc (lordosis or reversed "C" curve, like the neck) in your lower back. This is called the "weight lifter's arch."
- Knees are slightly bent to provide shock absorption.

Note: Again, it is important to note that all of the essentials work together. These are the curves evaluated, corrected, and maintained by a trained chiropractor (see essential 2) in order to maintain maximum nerve supply for maximized living.

Note: Perfect posture should be maintained during *all* stretches and exercises. Any exercise or stretch that calls for a disruption of posture is unhealthy or you are doing it wrong.

Quick Sets Give More for Less

Research shows that exercising only one or two times per week gives you all the benefits of *no exercise*. Frankly, then, it is just a waste of your time and energy. So when it comes to exercise you must always ask yourself, "Will I keep it up?"

As unfair as it may seem, the body is very much of a "What have you done for me lately?" organism. Starting and stopping exercise programs or infrequently exercising does you no good. Actually, it does more harm than good.

In weight resistance training, utilizing similar principles to SURGE training allows you to work an individual body part in as little as three minutes. Plus, these Quick Sets are radically more effective than typical, longer exercise sessions.

By performing Quick Sets, you are able to create significant changes in the composition (body-fat percentage and muscle tone) of a body part within three minutes. These routines can be used to increase the intensity of your workouts, shorten your workout times, and very safely speed up your results. They are designed so that anyone

Losing weight
without increasing
muscle means
only that you'll
fit in a
smaller coffin.

can perform them and make great changes on any level. Whether you are simply trying to lose the spare tire or pick up an Olympic medal, Quick Sets will work for you.

For the purpose of fitness, there are only eight body parts to consider: Chest, biceps, triceps, shoulders, abdominals, back/lats, legs (which include quads, hams, glutes, inner/outer thighs), and calves. By exercising with squats or lunges, you can actually hit your hamstrings, quads, the glutes (butt), and inner and outer thighs (typical trouble spots for women) all with one exercise.

Hit each body part once per week, and you'll only invest about twenty-four minutes to get in great shape! Add that to the thirty-six minutes of cardiovascular SURGE training, and you get maximum exercise benefits for a *total elapsed time of sixty minutes—one hour—per week!*

Types of Resistance Exercises

Leg Exercises
- Squat
- One-legged squat
- Lunges
- Straight-leg dead lift
- Dumbbell hamstring curl
- Calf raise

Upper Body Exercises
- Flye press
- Dumbbell curl
- Inclined dumbbell flye press
- Hammer curl
- Dumbbell flye
- Inclined dumbbell curl
- Triceps pushdown
- One-arm standing triceps extension
- One-arm bent triceps extension
- Dumbbell shoulder press
- Reverse-grip pulldown
- Lateral flye
- Front-grip pulldown

High body fat-to-muscle ratios negatively affect organ function, hormone balances, immune control, brain activity, and blood chemistry.

Your muscles were created for digging, climbing, and wrestling, not simply cracking open a soda.

MaximizedLivingMakeover.com

SPECIAL EXERCISE TIPS

for women, including pregnant women—watch the video and read the latest from Dr. Sheri Lerner.

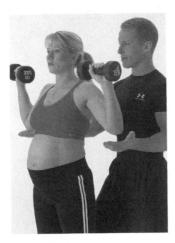

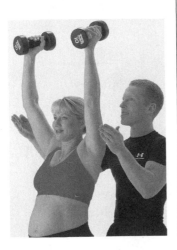

- Bent-rear deltoid flye
- One-arm dumbbell row
- Abdominal exercises
- Bent-knee leg raise
- Side hip raise

Learning More about Dumbbell Shoulder Press

This is a critical exercise for women, as they tend to be weak in this area. It is something that you have to work on because shoulders are really important to maintaining good posture. You start with your palms in and rotate on the way up. You always want to keep a little bit of a bend at the top, never locking the arms. Breathe in on the way down. Breathe out on the way up. Maintain good posture. Again, you do not want your head to go forward. We see a lot of neck injuries coming into chiropractors' offices because of heads going forward when you are lifting over your head.

Resistance exercise is a cornerstone of Maximized Living. Be sure to visit www.MaximizedLivingMakeover.com to:

- See pictures, explanations, *and actual video demonstrations* of all the exercises mentioned above.
- Get specific suggestions for optimum combinations for women and men.
- See sample quicksets that target the upper and lower body.

Types of Quick Sets

Decline Set

- Pick one exercise and do it for eight to twelve repetitions until failure.
- Rest for five to six seconds.
- Lower the weight five to twenty pounds and do the same exercise again for six to eight repetitions until failure.
- Rest five to six seconds.
- Lower the weight five to twenty pounds again and do another six to eight repetitions until failure.

Pause Set (You will experience the benefits of Pause Sets in the Maximized Living Intermediate Makeover Challenge.)

- Pick one exercise and do it for eight to twelve repetitions until failure.
- Rest five to six seconds.
- Using the same weight, do the exercise again until failure.
- Rest five to six seconds
- Repeat this process until you cannot do the exercise for more than one to two repetitions.

Monster Set

A Monster Set is when, after performing an exercise on one body part, instead of resting, you immediately perform an exercise on *another* body part. The other body part should be one that was not used while exercising the first body part. For example: combine chest and biceps, or quadriceps and hamstrings.

Monster Sets are combined with Decline or Pause Sets so you can get a tremendously effective workout done in a very short amount of time. For example, after you perform a Pause Set with the incline flye press for your chest, you can immediately begin performing a Decline Set with hammer curls for your biceps.

Tips for a Maximized Quick Set Workout

1. *Warm up! Warm up! Warm up!*: Do five to ten minutes of stretching and one to two warm-up sets of twelve to fifteen reps with very light weight before beginning your exercises. Stretching, warming up the muscles, and adding weight slowly will drastically reduce or eliminate your chance of injury.

2. Beginners, or people attempting just to maintain or develop some strength and muscle tone, should perform only one routine a week for lower body and one for upper body.

3. Upper-body workouts can be split in half by both men and women to make them shorter and more time efficient.

> Perfect posture should be maintained during *all* stretches and exercises.

> Starting and stopping exercise programs or infrequently exercising does more harm than good.

MaximizedLivingMakeover.com

Special exercise tips for
ELITE TRAINING
Watch the video from
Dr. Ben Lerner.

For example, chest, biceps, and triceps can be exercised separately from back, shoulders, and abdominals.

4. Change your routines around every week or month so you do not get bored and so that you avoid plateaus due to your body becoming accustomed to your routine.

Tip: If you are suffering injuries, regularly feeling excessively sore, physically exhausted, or burned out, then you are overtraining. When this happens, take an extra day or days off and/or lower the intensity of the workouts for a week or two. These signs also mean that you need more hydration and more intake of foods that reduce and/or neutralize acids in the body.

Final Tips for Essential 4: The Best Time to Exercise

The best time to exercise is first thing in the morning on an empty stomach. Why? Because exercising after resting and fasting through the night has extra benefits. Your growth hormone (HGH) levels are higher, your testosterone levels are at their highest, insulin is at its lowest (and that aids with fat burning), and it "turns on" your metabolism. If you eat prior to working out, any high amounts of fat will impede the release of HGH. It is important, however, to eat a post-workout meal within the first sixty minutes after exercising. We call this the "magic window" of time, as carbohydrates are absorbed by the body in the ideal fashion to help you recover.

Note: However, that ingesting high amounts of sugar after a workout will impair HGH response. So watch out for sports drinks!

A good recovery meal should contain about 25 grams of protein and 25 grams of carbohydrates for the optimal synergy meal. A protein powder mixed into a fruit smoothie is an easy way to accomplish this.

> You can create significant changes in the composition of a body part within three minutes.

Maximized Living Utilizing Essential 4 = the Ultimate Body in One Hour Per Week!

- 4 SURGE workouts per week = 12 minutes of exercise with 36 minutes of total elapsed time

  PLUS

- 3 minutes of exercise for each of the 8 basic body parts = 24 minutes of total elapsed time

- 1 hour of total time invested each week to get in great shape!

That's truly Maximized Living! Now, what's your excuse?

TAKE A STEP FORWARD!

1. The most important element you need for survival is oxygen. Carefully evaluate yourself for the signs of poor oxygen acquisition. Be sure to take the online oxygen inventory at www.MaximizedLivingMakeover.com. It will help you!

2. The benefits of exercise are too numerous and significant to ignore. Start moving today! Exercise doesn't have to take long or be boring—and it should never hurt.

3. Surge Training makes it possible to give your body the movement it needs in just 12 minutes a week. It's even better than aerobic exercise—and much faster. If you haven't consulted with your physician on starting an exercise program, schedule an appointment today.

4. Building muscle mass through resistance (weight) training has many benefits. Go to www.MaximizedLiving-Makeover.com to see pictures and videos of exercises that will not only improve your strength, but also help your balance, flexibility, and function.

> The best time to exercise is first thing in the morning on an empty stomach.

> It is important, however, to eat a post-workout meal within the first sixty minutes after exercising.

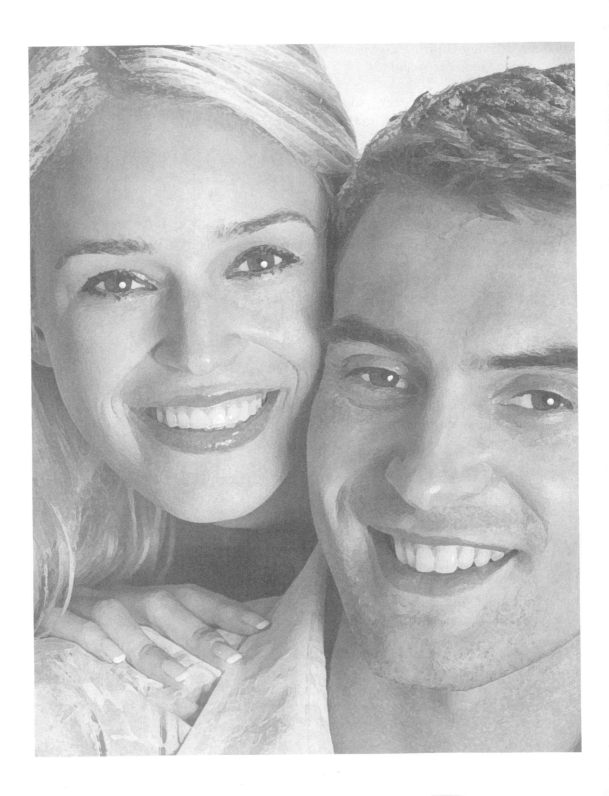

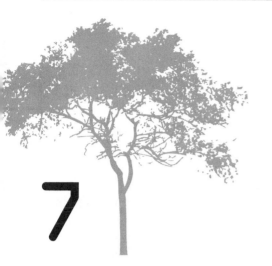

7

ESSENTIAL 5:
Maximize Peace and Relationships

Essential 5: maximize peace and relationships, may seem out of place when you consider the first four essentials, but it is just as important a component to achieve Maximized Living. Maximized Living is the total package. It is about the body, yes. It is about the mind and central nervous system, of course. But it is much more than that. True Maximized Living encompasses and benefits *all* aspects of your life, and that must include your emotions, relationships and the amount of peace you have.

Maximized Living isn't about prescribing or staying away from medications. It isn't about marriage counseling or therapy. It is about finding ways to maximize the total package of your life.

In today's American society and beyond, the majority of us are overwhelmed, overstressed, overstimulated, and overfed. We quite simply go overboard on just about everything. On the flip side, we are undisciplined, undermotivated, and unable to move forward in important areas of our lives.

Maximized
Living
Makeover
.com

READ

MaximizedLivingMakeover.com

WHAT'S
EATING YOU?
PART 1
A special report by Dr. Greg Loman on the connection between peace and heart disease.

> Maximized Living is about finding ways to maximize the total package of your life.

WHAT'S
EATING YOU?
PART 2
A special report by Dr. Charles Majors on the connection between stress and cancer.

Ten years ago, no one had ever heard of serotonin. Now, with the advent of antidepressants (selective serotonin re-uptake inhibitors or SSRIs) and epidemic use of these toxic drugs, most people are familiar with the term. As the name suggests, SSRIs work by preventing the neurons in the brain from reabsorbing the neurotransmitter serotonin. Essentially, they shut down a portion of the brain, and the brain is not a good organ to play with. Therefore, the negative side effects are enormous.

While there is no definitive way to determine what the "normal" levels of serotonin should be, what is clear is that people are burning out, damaging, and running out of these neurotransmitters due to being under a continual state of mental and chemical pressure from a rushed, stressed-out society that is hopped up on caffeine and sugar!

Every negative stimulus or emotion causes neurotransmitter stress and pain somewhere in your body. Therefore, if your overbooked schedule and tension don't get you, your Starbucks addiction will. The combination is even more toxic.

In our high-tech, high-chemical, fast-paced new millennium, we're running out of neurotransmitters fast.

Therefore, peace of mind and great relationships—the basics of essential 5—are very much connected to all of the five essentials. Toxicity, nerve function, nutrition, and fitness have clear connections to brain function and even emotional wellness. Additionally, much of relationship success pivots on the energy levels, health, moods, and well-being of the people connected in relationships. In all areas of life, including emotional and relational ones, Maximized Living application is about being proactive, not reactive (as opposed to antidepressants, for example, which are a quick-fix reaction with long-term, disastrous consequences).

The focus of Maximized Living isn't just about fixing what's already broken—bodies, minds, spirits, and relationships. Ideally, Maximized Living helps you build a life that never becomes broken. If it's already broken, Maximized Living offers you the best chance of being able

> Antidepressants shut down a portion of the brain, and the brain is not a good organ to play with.

to lay down the building blocks of a firm foundation to fix it. By building on new, healthy essentials, we give ourselves the best chance at healing and—most importantly—stopping the damage before it ever occurs.

Maximized Living teaches principles of peace and time management, and it lets you in on the secrets for building muscle-bound (strong) relationships. The goal is to prevent crisis, reduce debilitating stress, and help people regain control over their schedules and their lives. As a result, we hope to make your doctors, pharmacists, and psychiatrists a little poorer, if not broke—unless, of course, they want to start teaching Maximized Living.

The Life-Management Component: An Essential for the Maximized Life

Most people would probably like to be rich and famous. But before you could really make an informed decision on whether you would want to be a well-known athlete or famous billionaire, you would need to spend a day in their shoes. If they're stressed out, on spouse number three, and their kids are in and out of jail—being rich and famous wouldn't look nearly as appealing. You probably wouldn't want their life, no matter how good it looked from the outside.

Without peace of mind and strong relationships, neither life nor health can be maintained at maximum levels. With six of the top ten medications sold today being prescribed for depression, half of marriages continuously ending in divorce, children failing to thrive, and stressed, rushed lives being reported by practically all U.S. citizens, clearly we're failing big time at essential 5. Truth be told, if you can't make this essential a reality, not a whole lot else matters.

Bottom Line of Essential 5
We have to do something about our stress and how we relate to people to succeed at Maximized Living.

The idea of "managing" stress is similar to the idea of managing or treating symptoms and illness. The medical model treats unwanted health or disease with pills, vitamins,

> Much of relationship success pivots on the energy levels, health, moods, and well-being of the people connected in relationships.

> By building on new, healthy essentials, we give ourselves the best chance at healing and—most importantly— stopping the damage before it ever occurs.

weight loss, surgery—basically not much more than "magic" potions and leeches. This model of health and fitness has been a painful failure. Stress management in this medical model is treating stress with positive thinking or Prozac. Again, that model has been agonizing and unsuccessful.

The Maximized Living Model is never about fighting the darkness; it's about turning on the light.

Building peace is better than managing stress, and building strong relationships is way better than fixing broken ones.

Essential 5 is the life-management component of Maximized Living. Life management includes the following:

- Gaining new perspectives on life
- Getting control of your time
- Using the time you have more efficiently and effectively

When you get a grip on these three, they will afford you more than a sufficient amount of quality time and energy to be poured into your most important relationships.

Creating peace and strong relationships does not begin by changing everyone and every circumstance surrounding you. Switching locations, jobs, or spouses is typically *not* the answer to maintaining peace and healthy relationships. While the grass always seems greener (or in this case, more peaceful) in someone else's yard, occupation, or relationship, once you get over there, over *there* becomes *here*. As the saying goes, "Wherever you go, there you are." Peace of mind and better associations start and end with you. When *you* change, the atmosphere around you changes.

It is easy to blame outside influences for your anxiety and stress. Blaming things outside of your life for what goes on inside of you and your life is self-defeating. It implies that there's nothing *you* can do about it. That's a victim mentality, and you never want to give in to that kind of rationalizing. You're not simply controlled by your circumstances or your genes and fated for anxiety, depression, stress, and a dysfunctional family. You have influence. You have power for change.

You have a lot to say about your present and your future. Sometimes it's just a matter of gaining a new perspective on the circumstances and relationships around you.

Gaining New Perspectives

The first part of life management is changing your perspective. The goal here is to make the virtual leap from the fish bowl into the ocean and to go from being stuck behind a tree at the bottom of the mountain to looking out from its peak. If you change your perspective or vantage point in life, then you begin see and handle life much differently.

In his book *Man's Search for Meaning*, Holocaust survivor Dr. Victor Frankl described life in a concentration camp. He marched for miles everyday in one-size-fits-all wooden shoes, in ragged unwashed clothes, in frozen temperatures, working at hard meaningless tasks, and with only thin soup and moldy bread to eat. Additionally, he lived in a shack with no temperature control and a leaking roof, and he slept on a hard wooden bench with multiple other men. To make matters even more desperate, on the day Dr. Frankl was brought to the concentration camp, his family was taken and murdered and all his possessions were stolen from him.

Through it all, Dr. Frankl kept a victorious outlook. He realized that in these death camps, those who died (that were not murdered) were the ones who could see nothing but their overwhelming pain and suffering. Dr. Frankl determined to keep his circumstances—tragic as they were—in perspective. Despite all the odds, he not only survived, but also he kept a positive attitude. He teaches us that when all is seemingly taken away, you still have one thing left: your right to choose your perspective and, thus, your attitude about your circumstances.

If you are struggling to keep a good perspective against seemingly overwhelming circumstances in your life, here are five steps for improving your perspective and working toward the goal of Maximized Living.

> Without peace of mind and strong relationships, neither life nor health can be maintained at maximum levels.

> When *you* change, the atmosphere around you changes.

Five Steps for Improving Your Perspective on Life

1. Recognize your value
2. Discover your UTP: Unique Talent Proposition
3. Find a Higher Purpose
4. Create a Personal Value System
5. Dismiss Results and Reactions

What do each of these five steps mean? Some are easier than others to understand right off the bat. But even the easiest to accept at face value can be difficult, at times, to do. Here's a deeper look at these five crucial steps to gaining a new perspective on your life.

1. Recognize your value.

Whether it seems like it or not, you matter. You matter to history, you matter to the world, you matter to the purpose you were created to serve, and you're needed by the people around you. You have tremendous value. Yes, you!

Your value or worth is not determined by image. In a world full of pain, confusion, and aimless materialism, your occupation, your finances, and your possessions might determine your position or image, but they have nothing to do with your worth.

Once you've labeled yourself, you devalue yourself. If you call yourself poor, short, fat, ugly, divorced, addicted, lazy, a procrastinator, not a morning person, not an achiever, not a reader, a poor leader, old, arthritic, nonenergetic, and so on, you start buying into and creating a destiny you weren't designed for. Labeling has caused people to feel ashamed, defeated, and inadequate because they've been judged. They actually program themselves, or allow themselves to be programmed by those around them, to think of themselves as bad, unacceptable, abnormal, and less capable than all the other people on the planet.

This low self-esteem, poor-self-image mind-set that marks you as "unworthy" is faulty programming, but you can change all that—starting today. That's the great thing about life. It is not about the past; it's about the present and the future. In fact, the past has nothing to do with what you can do today or what you can accomplish tomorrow and for the remainder of your "tomorrows." (And with Maximized Living, you'll have a lot of them!)

Your worth cannot be counted in power, fame, fortune, or what you did or didn't do yesterday. It's based solely on the value of your uniqueness and all of your incredible potential. When a baby is born, it holds no job and has no possessions, yet its value is indescribable and its potential limitless. And here's the great part that most people don't realize: the value and potential that you were born with don't leave or depreciate as you age!

Isn't that awesome? Think about it. Nothing is more common than people who seemingly have everything, yet because they've put their value in those things they lose sight of their worth and therefore who they are. They end up from our perspective (there's that word again) on top of the world. But from their perspective, they're miserable.

On the other hand, many clergy, teachers, civic servants, charity workers, missionaries, and others who serve those around them—though they have very little in the way of fame, money, power, or possessions—feel a deep sense of value and live incredibly fulfilling lives. What they don't accumulate in the social image bank account, they make up for with their investment in self-worth.

2. Discover your UTP: unique talent proposition.

There's a common mistaken belief that most Americans have been taught since babyhood that you can be anything you want to be. Unfortunately, that's just not true. If you're five feet, four inches tall, slow, and can't jump, you're most likely not going to ever make a professional football or basketball team. Similarly, if you struggle in math and, in fact, hate it, you will not make a good accountant—and why would you want to become one?

You can't be anything you want to be, but the great news is you can be everything you were born to be. In the first step to gaining a new perspective on your life, you recognized that you have value. In this second step, you learn to recognize your unique skills and talents. What do you have a passion for? What skills, professions, or games

You're not simply controlled by your circumstances or your genes and fated for anxiety, depression, stress, and a dysfunctional family.

> The first part of life management is changing your perspective.

come naturally to you? What work or job descriptions do you tend to excel at more then others? As you investigate these three questions, you begin to discover your talent. And your talents and skills are your unique talent proposition.

Another myth that we've all been sold is that we should spend most of our time improving our weaknesses. While improving areas that are holding you back is important, the best thing you can actually do is spend time strengthening your strengths. It's like a frog that determines that he is going to learn to fly in order to get across a pond instead of just hopping over it. It's a pretty big pond, and despite his best efforts to fly, all he does is feebly flap his legs and fall into the water. The frog simply will never be good at flying, no matter how long he spends trying to overcome this "weakness."

Instead, he'd get over the pond much more quickly and efficiently if he practiced his hopping—something he was designed to do in the first place! Hopping is his forte, and when he improves his hop (rather than wishing he could grow wings), he maximizes his unique talent proposition.

Maybe that was kind of a silly illustration, but you get our point. Don't try and turn the areas where your talent (on a scale of 1 to 10) is a 2 into a 4 or 5, when you'd be much better served by turning the areas where you're already a 6 or 7 into 9 and 10. Plus, when you work in the areas of your strengths, you enjoy it. It doesn't feel like work. That's the key to determining your passions: do what you love, and do it the very best that you can.

3. Find a higher purpose.

Now that you know your value and are concentrating on strengthening your unique skills and talents, it's time to make sure you are doing these things for a higher purpose.

The word *purpose* means "the object for which you exist."

With your valuable UTP in place, you can now discover your reason for living—the purpose you were called to serve. This doesn't mean (necessarily) that you change jobs, girlfriends or boyfriends, or move to Sedona, Arizona. It does mean, however, that you stop doing what you believe you should, ought, or must do and start doing what you were born to do. When you know you're doing something that is right, for the greater good, and something that adds value to the world, you're a hard person to upset, depress, or stop. It also gives you passion, which makes you an exciting person to be around.

In determining your true purpose, you have to self-examine and ask yourself some pretty important questions: What is the object for which I exist? Why was I born? Why do I exist at all? More specifically, you want to determine: What is my purpose as a parent? What is the purpose of my business? What is my purpose as a spouse, friend, or neighbor?

Defining your purpose is like setting a compass; it gives you direction. The more time you spend checking your compass, the more assurance you have that you will stay on the selected path and get ever closer to your selected destination. We all have things we're responsible for and have to do. Yet, if you keep living a life that is just about paying the bills and doing what you gotta do, you've lost your purpose—or you never discovered it in the first place. Your purpose keeps you on course. What makes Maximized Living so exciting is the thrill of the mission that your purpose fulfills.

4. Create a personal value system.

When you have determined your purpose in life, you then establish a set of values to guide you. People with higher purpose possess higher values. The famous psychiatrist Abraham Maslow created a "hierarchy of needs." At the bottom of his pyramid, someone or something is simply roaming the earth looking to meet their basic needs of water, food, shelter, and self-preservation. At the top, where higher beings belong, the search that consumes life is for significance or purpose.

We live in a world that Maslow essentially described as a "rodent culture." (Why do you think we describe our busy lives as a "rat race"?) Our culture has become a place where people live, work, and scurry to meet their lower needs with little thought of significance—their ultimate

> When all is taken away, you still have one thing left: your right to choose your perspective.

> Once you've labeled yourself, you devalue yourself. If you call yourself poor, short, fat, ugly, divorced, addicted, lazy, a procrastinator, you start buying into and creating a destiny you weren't designed for.

MaximizedLivingMakeover.com

WHAT DOES SUCCESS LOOK LIKE TO YOU?

Write your thoughts.

need. Sadly, we've become a WIFM—What's in it for me?—society. Our current culture, using Maslow's metaphor, has become a bunch of lower beings fighting for what's theirs. With your purpose and values intact, you will rise to the top of the pyramid, literally living "above it all."

True success is found in significance, living a purposeful life using your UTP to make an impact in the lives of people and adding to, not taking from, the world. If purpose is like a compass, a personal value system is true north. It turns the navigational compass into a moral compass. Without a moral compass, you find yourself at any given point by chance, never going in a straight line, never being on any particular course. Never sacrifice your values for your needs.

5. Dismiss results and reactions.

Nothing sets you up more for emotional failure than when your life slips away from expressing your uniqueness, fulfilling your purpose, and living within your value system. All of this creates an internal conflict that psychologists can ultimately have a field day discussing and charge you a fortune to treat. This deep internal struggle is the emotional plight of the new millennium, as people in today's world do what they can to fit in and keep up. In the process, they only lose themselves.

In our attempt to please people and get results in our work, we can lose sight of or completely abandon all that we've discussed. When you're on track, however, you are not affected by results or the opinion of others. Serve the purpose, not the results. Stick to your value system and let results take care of themselves. Just keep following your compass. You're better off taking it slow and heading in the right direction than heading fast—the wrong way.

If you're certain you are operating according to higher (not rodent) values, and someone's not happy with you, the problem probably lies with them. This doesn't take away from your responsibility to get along with those who love and depend on you. It just means you can keep some grip on your emotional responses when they don't understand. By living according to the principles we've discussed, you'll still have a sense of peace even when people aren't happy

> The great thing about life is that it's not about the past; it's about the present and the future.

with you or the results aren't there. You will still know your value, understand your uniqueness, maintain your values, and understand your purpose. If you have broken some of the rules, well, we all make mistakes. You'll correct what you can do better next time, right? Mistakes are common, but they do not define you. You're valuable. In fact, you're invaluable to this world. In all of the earth, there is no one else exactly like you. When you remember that and line up all the components you've been taught in this book, that's when you'll be well on your way to maximized living.

Depression and Maximized Living

We asked an expert, Gwen Olsen, author of *Confessions of an Rx Drug Pusher*, about the real cause of depression and what could be done outside of relying on antidepressant medication. Here's how she replied:

> Because we know stress can affect brain chemistry, it is entirely plausible that emotions are often responsible for the low serotonin and norepinephrine levels found in people suffering with depression.
>
> Depression has been defined by some psychologists as 'anger turned inward.' Many circumstances can predispose an individual to depression, including loss of a parent, emotional neglect or trauma experienced in childhood, or stressful life experiences in general (for example, death, divorce, job loss or other financial stress).
>
> However, there are a host of other possibilities that could account for this biochemical phenomenon, including low thyroid function, heavy metals toxicity, nutritional deficiencies, hormonal imbalances, candidiasis, blood sugar imbalances, environmental toxin or chemical exposure, environmental or food allergens, infectious disease, and both the use of and withdrawal from CNS (central nervous system) depressant drugs (such as narcotic painkillers, sleep aids, antianxiety drugs, antidepressants).
>
> All of these complex concerns are best managed through building function and healing by addressing their associate

When a baby is born, it holds no job and has no possessions; yet, its value is indescribable and its potential limitless.

You can't be anything you want to be, but the great news is you can be everything you were born to be.

VICTIM
TO VICTOR

Write down the one step you can take today—and gain inspiration from the steps others just like you are taking.

essentials for Maximized Living rather than just writing them essentials for Maximized Living rather than just writing them off as something to be "managed" by yet another complicating chemical entity.

As for the validity of depression being classified as a "mental illness," the well-known adage, "Sound body—sound mind" reveals a basic simple truth. That is, depression is commonly intertwined with a vast number of diverse conditions and illnesses.

Uncovering the origin of potential imbalances can be a powerful tool in selecting effective natural and holistic approaches to emotional healing. In addition to heavy metals and mercury toxicity, testing is available to identify imbalances and deficiencies in levels of amino acids, food and environmental allergens, melatonin, cortisol in the adrenal glands, digestive function including measurement of Candida albicans, fatty acids, glucose and insulin, female hormonal panels, and thyroid imbalances. All of these issues can cause depression and mood disorders, overlooked by psychiatric evaluations where physical causes are ignored. See your Maximized Living doctor for help!

Life-Management Mastery—
the Key to Less Stress (and Happier Relatives)

Pressure or stress is a way of life. But you can reduce it and even aim to eliminate it, rather than simply always trying to operate in "crisis management." Reprogramming the way you respond to pressure is great, but reducing the stress you live with is even better.

You can reduce stress by replacing it with peace. This is more than thinking positively. Peace of mind is not simply passive. It's actively living in such a way that reduces the amount of turmoil and stress-producing circumstances that become insurmountable when flying blind.

Most, if not all, of the trouble you find yourself in, you created. You may not see it. That's why they call them "blind spots"—you're blind to them. For example (and it's a scary

When you work in the areas of your strengths, it doesn't feel like work.

one if you've ever experienced it), an eighteen-wheeler can be hidden when you look in a one-inch piece of rearview mirror. It's invisible to the eye, but it's definitely still there, and it brings death if you do not become aware of it before you change lanes.

If you practice your paces until you become a maximized-living and life-management "black belt," the potential dangers to your relationships and peace of mind lessen. As they say in the marriage world, "If you want to stay out of court, keep courting." In life management, you should always court good health, finances, friends, family, peace of mind, and all that it takes to set yourself up for maximized living so that you don't become like most folks—emotionally, physically, relationally, and financially in divorce court.

One big practical way you can reduce stress and keep peace of mind and relationships is to get organized.

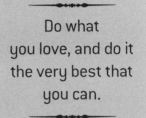

Do what you love, and do it the very best that you can.

Life Management 101: The Art of the "To-Do" List (Write It Down)

You stand back and look at the mountain you have to climb on your own. You see nothing but thick brush, a dense forest of trees, large sharp rocks, unprotected drop-offs, and no visible trail of any kind. Oh yeah, and there's a torrential downpour. In fact, as you look up you see that somewhere around midway toward the top, the rain turns into snow and a vicious blizzard. You are ill prepared to take this mountain on in this condition, yet you know that you have no choice but to start climbing.

For many, this is what their week looks like every Sunday night, inducing the question: "How will I ever make it to the top?" or, in other words, through the week! Once the week starts, it's not much different than the mountain portrayed above: poor visibility, uncertain footing, stressful climbs, a rugged climate, substantial effort, dangerous turns, and no help.

Now imagine that you went to the other side of the mountain, and there in front of you is a clearly laid-out path with handrails, rest stop cafes with food and plug-in

MaximizedLivingMakeover.com

5 LIFE-TRANSFORMING TOPICS

Go in-depth with the five steps. Get to know more on these life-transforming topics.

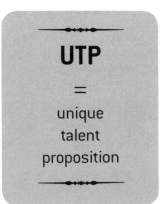

heaters, and plenty of experienced people ready to help. There's still quite a climb to accomplish, but now there's no doubt you'll get there more peacefully.

In this illustration, you're seeing the difference between someone without a clear, written plan and someone with one. If you look at your day or week—your personal mountain—and have nothing written out or planned, then it feels enormous. (Remember, negative feelings about your week equals pain somewhere in your body and serotonin burnout.)

Yet if you take the same exact mountain (week) and write out exactly what needs to be done and when, it suddenly seems very climbable. And if you have strong relationships—you usually have guides (people who love you) who will help. With a clear written list, there might still be a whole lot to do, and it may be stressful still, but when you're feeling strongly about your ability to conquer your list, that stress won't conquer you.

Perhaps the most painful, serotonin-depleting life-management mistake you can make is what we call "memory management." Memory management is simply trying to remember everything you have to do. It's the most literal interpretation there is of making mountains out of molehills! Your brain wasn't built to keep all the details of your week in it without missing or forgetting something. (Remember the frog that was determined to fly?) If you keep attempting to manage your schedule this way, you'll make it feel like Mt. Everest. As a result, you'll be constantly stressed out and extremely ineffective.

There are two necessary terms we use to show you how to best lay out your path in order to climb it more easily and successfully.

1. The written to-do list is a written list that let's you see exactly what to do and eliminates memory management.
2. The war plan is when you convert the to-do list into an action plan. You take what has to be done and give it a specific day, time, and length in order to accomplish it without worry.

The Written To-Do List

The written to-do list is simple and self-explanatory. It's Life Management 101: "Write it down." Nothing should be stored only in the mental files. Make out a list at the beginning of each week either in a planner, electrical planner, a computer file marked "to-do for the week of_____," a calendar, or do it "old school" in a notebook. This is an absolute minimum for living with any degree of success or sanity.

The War Plan

Make no mistake about it—you're at war. You're in a daily war fighting against disease, debt, emotional turmoil, weight gain, shrinking muscles, divorce and failed relationships. If you're a parent, you're also fighting against all of the enemies your children have to face that would block their health and future. And for many reading this right now, the enemies listed above aren't even the half of it!

Some would call our organizational method for maximized living a game plan, but some of life's battles are just too brutal to call them a game, so we've labeled it the war plan to help you understand how important this is as a tool to fight off some of your stress-inducing enemies. No matter how badly you want to win, you can't win a game, much less a war, without a strategic plan of attack. Without a war plan, you will lose the battles and in the end, the whole war. As it's often said, "The will to win is not nearly as important as the will to prepare to win."

The war plan is your to-do list broken up into what days and times each task is going to happen, along with how much time you've designated to "git 'er done." There is always enough time to get the important things done, but it is often the immediate that consumes our days, leaving the important tasks gathering dust on a back shelf somewhere as we swear we'll get around to them someday soon. The problem never truly is that there is not enough time; the problem is that there is not enough *time management*.

A vital part of essential 5 is strong relationships. Working out the quality and the quantity of time and communication necessary to build strength requires an expertise in weekly

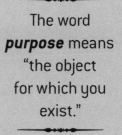

The word *purpose* means "the object for which you exist."

MaximizedLivingMakeover.com

RECOGNIZING YOUR VALUE

What is the biggest challenge you face in recognizing your value? Get support from others who are overcoming the same challenges.

> Stop doing what you believe you should, ought, or must do, and start doing what you were born to do.

planning. While a strong relationship isn't solely dependent on time, it also won't happen without it.

Whether you've taken the time to recognize it or not, you have multiple areas of your life that need to be done well. Like a cat, you have at least nine lives that need attention each week to flourish—and some people have even more. Let me show you what we mean.

Your Nine Lives
1. Mental health life
2. Family life
3. Personal health and fitness life
4. Financial life
5. Purpose life
6. Recreational life
7. Relationship with friends and coworkers life
8. Community obligations life
9. Education and personal growth life

If even one of the above doesn't thrive, it typically impedes the success of all the others. If you're financially fit but physically sick, you can end up losing mental health, hurting your family, not fulfilling your purpose, and so on. No wonder you're stressed and overwhelmed. You have at least nine lives that you're living! (Does that make you tired just thinking about it? Are you ready for a nap now?)

These lives are there whether you want them or not, and all of them deserve your attention and need the strongest war plan possible. Like the scary, solitary mountain climb we described before, if you don't have a clear, safe path and strategy, life's going to hurt. On the other hand, with a plan in place it's not hard to keep it all together.

Putting the Plan Together—Creating Solid Yellow Boxes

Busy, successful people can stay focused. They compartmentalize their time so they can get multiple things done better than many people can get *one* thing done. They are able to focus. Focus in a war means you can't be looking at or thinking about something else. Your total energies are centered on the battle at hand. Being distracted can be the difference between success and failure, life or death. When you're putting time into an area of your life, it also needs focused energy. We call this present time consciousness or "up time" (UT).

What you need to do as you formulate your personal war plan is draw lines around each one of your lives. Think of it like this: when you are driving, if there is a dotted yellow line, you can pass or cross over into the other lane. However, if there is a solid yellow line, you cannot pass and you cannot cross over. Others cannot pass or cross over either.

If you paint solid yellow lines around each of your lives and the to-do's they contain, other lives cannot pass or cross over. If you then visualize these lives as solid yellow boxes and put them into your to-do list, you're focused and the time spent is all UT. When you operate within one "boxed" life, all six sides are solid yellow and you stay completely present-time conscious to the task at hand in that box. You can't step, look, or see outside a solid yellow box. You're forced to stay focused on what's in it and only what's in it.

The box causes you to completely direct your attention to your work, your spouse, your kids, or your golf game so that you're thinking of nothing else. Nothing is less effective then the man who thinks about having sex with his wife the whole time he's at work and who thinks about work the whole time he's having sex with his wife!

Maintaining solid, six-walled boxes makes you better at every one of your lives. Multitasking isn't really doing five things at once, because you can't think more than one thought at a time or do more than one thing at a time. Your ability to focus on a multitude of boxes in a brief window of time is a good definition of the new millennium multitasker.

> When you know you're doing something that is right, for the greater good, and something that adds value to the world, you're a hard person to upset, depress, or stop, and you're an exciting person to be around.

YOUR UTPs

Write down your UTP—what you were born to do—and be inspired by the UTP's of others. What is the object for which you exist? What is the reason you were born?

> When you have determined your purpose in life, you then establish a set of values to guide you.

Solid Yellow Box Examples

MONDAY

7:00–7:10 a.m. Fitness life—SURGE training

From 7:00–7:10 a.m. you put yourself in the yellow box of SURGE training.

9:00–1:00 p.m. Financial life

You put yourself in the yellow box of your chosen occupation. By focusing on your work and not your eight other lives, along with a dozen other distractions, you'll succeed and more than likely vastly improve your financial prospects. No other life is allowed in at that time. No personal calls, no exercise "breaks," no personal growth at that time. Do not look at an e-mail.

1:15–2:30 p.m. Lunch date with spouse

Here you put yourself in the yellow box of family life. Fully concentrate on your spouse during this time. Don't let colleagues intrude on your time. Don't answer your cell phone. Stay in your yellow box.

2:45–5:45 p.m. Financial life

6:30–9:15 p.m. Family life

From 6:00 until 9:15 each evening, there's a very impenetrable solid yellow family box. Again, you're in the box. This means relational time, not TV, cell phones, or Internet. That's quality UT. Plus, by making sure this time is penciled firmly in place consistently each day, it's also quantity UT. If you want strong relationships and healthy children who grow up to be healthy, productive successful adults, you need quality and quantity focused time.

9:15–10:00 p.m. Education and personal growth life

A book or computer program designed to advance learning in an area important to the advancement of your personal life. This could also be time for relaxation or going to sleep.

Not every minute has something in it, but ideally every life is scheduled. Sometimes it's nap life, but it's still scheduled. (I learned that one in kindergarten.) Certain lives happen every day, but others are strategically placed throughout the week so all that items on the written to-do list are checked off and done *well*.

Obviously, it doesn't always work out so perfectly. Sometimes a child wakes up during times designated for mental exercises (as seen at the end of essential 5) or an extremely urgent issue pops up that cannot be handled by the people who now help you in life. At those times, you have to practice flexibility. If lives cross over into other lanes or lives, as they occasionally will, try to remember the admonition, "That's life." Work to get past the issues and try to get everyone and everything back in their lanes as quickly as possible before there is an accident!

Unfortunately, a few times a year there are some traumatic, stressful five-lives pileups. But by getting back to healthy compartmentalization through the building of solid yellow boxes and proper delegation, you can usually manage to escape with only some minor damage.

Families: The Special Yellow Box

Lives are like the rows of flowers in a garden. They need nourishment and attention. If you have a family, time needs to be allotted for the whole family unit, individual time for each family member needs to be considered, and the kids' lives all need to be scheduled, too. Families need a variety of different "lives," just to interact with each other.

There are family date times, which are time spent together as a family (*not* watching TV). You also need to box in date times with each child—and your spouse. Date times are fun or organized teaching times that are one on one, spending time together. Children also have activities that have to be scheduled into your lives, as well as organized for them to also start living maximized lives. These may include sports teams, homework, music lessons, games, parties, and personal growth time.

> If purpose is like a compass, a personal value system is true north. It turns the navigational compass into a moral compass.

Husbands and wives need to consult with each other to see how the time can be spent most equitably each week in order for family member to feel like their needs—especially the needs of the couple relationship—are being met. Husbands, ask your wives what they need from you, and what they think the kids need from you. Women tend to understand the emotional needs of the family better then men. Plus, the fact remains, "If momma ain't happy, nobody's happy."

Wives, on the other hand, need to respect their husband's mission. If you have a husband living on purpose, be good to your husband on purpose. The time that is not given to family should be free for your husband to use to provide and protect his family and to do his part to save the world. (Isn't that what all men feel hard-wired to do?)

Here's an example of what a child's solid yellow boxes for a week might look like:

Weekdays
4:00–5:30 p.m.
    School life, including schoolwork, reading, and educational videos

8:00–9:00 p.m.
    Play life (video game time)

Monday, Wednesday, Friday
3:00–4:00 p.m.
    Sports life (baseball practice)

Thursday nights, Saturday and Sunday afternoons
    Times vary: Family life

Saturdays
12:00–1:00 p.m.
    Hobby or music life (for example, piano lessons)

Remember, your child cannot be more organized or manage his life better than you do from the example you set!

> Never sacrifice your values for your needs.

> He who takes his time generally takes other people's time too.
> ~ *Anonymous*

Stepping into Greatness: Eliminate with a Chainsaw All That Doesn't Belong and You Can Sculpt Out a Future

Distractions are time thieves. They will rob precious time from you, your family, and your real purpose in life. More than likely more than anything else, you need to cut and delegate, cut and delegate, and then cut and delegate some more.

We live in an age of technology and industry where you can make money and get your taxes done while you sleep and go to Disney World. Do not accept that your life is irreparably busy. Lop off with a chainsaw anything that isn't necessary for the life of your dreams. If there is something that can't be cut now but that you don't want—what's the cutting-it-off plan? Make one!

Do not confuse contentment with complacency. It's easy to get comfortable. Because of this, many have lost jobs, lost families, and gained large waistlines. You're either growing or dying, so in order to keep the mission alive, plan daily and weekly growth. Many people look at guidelines for living as a lawful, dry, and boring existence. But they are not. Far from it! The life that is inspired is an exciting one. It is a life that goes beyond simple happiness to an inner sense of peace and fulfillment. It is the embodiment of Maximized Living.

Only the artist who's disciplined to practice his violin can truly play the vast harmonies and beautiful music throughout his life. The rest are doomed to play nothing. Schedule your time—and become free!

> Nothing sets you up more for emotional failure than when your life slips away from expressing your uniqueness, fulfilling your purpose, and living within your value system.

PERSONAL TIME CHART

Download the Personal Time Chart to schedule your time and become free.

PERSONAL TIME CHART

Morning / Afternoon				
Time:	Time:	Time:	Time:	Time:
Life:	Life:	Life:	Life:	Life:
Missionary Work:	Missionary Work:	Missionary Work:	Missionary Work:	Missionary Work:
Prosperity Time:	Prosperity Time:	Prosperity Time:	Prosperity Time:	Prosperity Time:

Afternoon / Evening				
Time:	Time:	Time:	Time:	Time:
Life:	Life:	Life:	Life:	Life:
Missionary Work:	Missionary Work:	Missionary Work:	Missionary Work:	Missionary Work:
Prosperity Time:	Prosperity Time:	Prosperity Time:	Prosperity Time:	Prosperity Time:

> You can still have a sense of peace, know your value, understand your uniqueness, maintain your values, and understand your purpose even when people aren't happy with you.

Exercising Your Emotions: Building Mental Muscle

In order to fully embrace essential 5: maximize peace and strong relationships, it's just as important to exercise your emotions as it is to exercise your body. Strong muscles afford us the opportunity to apply great resistance against the physical rigors of life. But what about mental muscles and emotional muscles? Have you exercised those regularly? By strengthening your mind and tending your heart (emotions), you prepare your will, fortify your resolve, and continue your journey to building peace. In the end, you'll be ready for anything.

Basic Emotion Exercises

Before a farmer plants, he prepares the soil. If we want to live to the fullest mentally, emotionally, spiritually, financially, and relationally, then we have to prepare our mental and emotional states. Like an athlete preparing for a big game, you have to "get in state." If we don't, then rather than managing the day's events, we allow the day's events and the people in them to manage us—to manage how we feel and how we react. Before we know it, we've become slaves to our circumstances and victims of our environment.

Situations and circumstances can be transcended if we learn how to prepare our minds. Honestly, even being prepared may not always be enough. You'll still get knocked down by circumstances in life. But if you are prepared, you'll get back up more quickly. A champion only has to get up one more time than he or she has been knocked down.

What can you do to get yourself in great mental and emotional shape? Practice emotional exercises like the Peace Triathlon.

Getting "In State" through the "Peace Triathlon"

What we talk about in Maximized Living is, again, not necessarily about managing mental and emotional stress. What we want to place emphasis on is creating and managing peace so that you don't get in a state of stress in the first place. The following emotional exercise is designed to maximize your emotional and mental preparedness for the day. The best time to perform this exercise is preferably first thing in the morning so that you are ready to take on your day.

The mind is most receptive to peace training in the morning, since the mind has the capacity to absorb more input at this time of day than any other. We call this exercise the mental and emotional Peace Triathlon, and the structure is as follows: Find a quiet part of your house where you can sit relaxed and undisturbed for fifteen minutes. Practice the following three parts of your Peace Triathlon:

1. Sit for five minutes in silence. Keep your mind empty; try to let no thoughts enter.

2. Spend the next five minutes on visualization. Focus on how you want to positively and proactively respond to the day's events. See yourself acting out mental and emotional control, especially in scheduled situations that you know could cause stress or tension.

3. Read for the last five minutes. Choose positive, inspiring, and empowering literature. For example, read a devotional, personal development book, inspiring biography, or the Bible.

Mistakes are common, but they do not define you.

> "Sound body—sound mind"

> Cherish your own vision and your dreams as they are the children of your soul, the blueprints of your ultimate achievements.
> ~ Napoleon Hill

> Everyone who got where he is had to begin where he was.
> ~ Robert Louis Stevenson

Intermediate Emotion Exercises: Sowing Your Seed, Feeding Your Attitude

Once the farmer has the soil ready, how can he realistically expect a crop if he never plants or sows any seeds? Likewise, how could any sane farmer believe that he can reap wheat, if all day long he's planting watermelon seeds? The human brain is no different than a field that has had its soil prepared, waiting on its seeds. The brain works off of the same laws of sowing and reaping. Sow a negative thought, and you reap a negative reality. Sow a positive thought, and you attract and enjoy the abundant, nutritious fruit of its harvest.

There's an old story that describes this well. An old Cherokee Indian was speaking to his grandson and said, "A fight is going on inside me. It is a terrible fight, and it is between two wolves. One is evil—he is anger, envy, sorrow, regret, greed, arrogance, self-pity, guilt, resentment, inferiority, lies, false pride, superiority, and ego. The other is good—he is joy, peace, love, hope, serenity, humility, kindness, benevolence, empathy, generosity, truth, compassion, and faith. This same fight is going on inside you, and inside every other person too."

The grandson thought about it for a long minute, and then asked his grandfather, "Which wolf will win?"

The old Cherokee replied simply, "The one you feed."

Quotes and affirmations are among the greatest positive seeds you can plant in your mind daily. Here is a sampling of quotations that will add strength to your mind and encouragement to your spirit:

> From the moment of your birth forward, you're allotted a very specific amount of time in your life. Your days are numbered.

> Strength does not come from winning. Your struggles develop your strengths. When you go through hardships and decide not to surrender, that is strength.
>
> ~ *Arnold Schwarzenegger, actor and governor of California*

> Our greatest weakness lies in giving up. The most certain way to succeed is always to try just one more time.
>
> ~ *Thomas Edison*

> The way to get started is to quit talking and begin doing.
>
> ~ *Walt Disney*

> The moment one definitely commits oneself, then providence moves too. A whole stream of events issues from the decision, raising in one's favor all manner of unforeseen incidents, meetings and material assistance, which no man could have dreamt would have come his way.
>
> ~ *William Murray, mountaineer*

> Life isn't about finding yourself. Life is about creating yourself.
>
> ~ *George Bernard Shaw*

Repeat these positive, affirming quotes and look for others to boost your spirits. Copy them onto small cards or sticky notes and post them where you will see them. Create your own positive phrases and get used to saying them to yourself. You can even say them out loud. Your kids might look at you funny, but they are good for them to hear too!

Elite Emotion Exercises:
Watering the Seed—Getting Upward Bound

The dominant thoughts and actions most people have throughout the day don't match up with the dreams they have for their lives. Elite exercises set the mental compass toward true north. If you have dreams, then count on

> One big practical way you can reduce stress, keep peace of mind, and maintain relationships is to get organized.

> Your brain wasn't built to keep all the details of your week in it without missing or forgetting something.

challenges. It's not often that the wind is at your back or that the path moves downhill. However, with your compass set in the right direction it won't matter which way the wind blows or how difficult the journey is. Eventually, you'll get there.

Now that you understand the importance of essential 5: maximize peace and strong relationships, ask yourself the following maximizing questions:

1. Do I see my desired future clearly?
2. Have I written down what I really want in life?
3. Do I tend to focus on the negative or the positive?
4. What is my vision for the future?
5. What is it that I really want out of life?

> The future you see is the future you get.
> ~ Robert G Allen, business, finance and motivational author

Setting the GPS

The best time to perform this action exercise is at the beginning of your day, preferably first thing in the morning. The mind is most receptive to peace training in the morning since the mind has the capacity to absorb more input at this time than any other.

This exercise is called "setting the GPS." Just like the new automobiles today have global positioning systems (GPS), so does the human brain. The great news (or it can also be the bad news) is that we set our own GPS. Our GPS can be a destructive one which is currently leading us right off a cliff, or it can be one that is accelerating us to unimaginable heights of success, happiness, health, and wealth. For this elite exercise, find a quiet part of your house where you can sit relaxed and undisturbed. Then set your GPS as follows:

1. Write down your three most important goals.
2. Write out your major definite purpose or goal in the present tense, as if it were already a reality.
3. Briefly describe what you are going to do today to achieve your goal. (Put it in a solid yellow box.)

> Your life is now! If you're not experiencing joy and health *now* and you're not working on and investing in your joy and health for later, you're blowing it!

4. Write your major problem or goal in the form of a question, such as "How can I lose twenty-five pounds?" or "How can I show that I am a more loving and caring spouse?"

5. Write out twenty answers to the above question.

Select one action from the above exercise to begin immediately. (Also put it in a solid yellow box.) Repeat this process every single day until it becomes a habit and is a permanent part of your brain's GPS circuitry.

Doing this exercise will help you work steadily toward the achievement of your goals throughout the day. You'll feel energized, hopeful, and powerful instead of fatigued, weak, and defeated.

Meditation/Relaxation:
Free Your Mind—the Rest Will Follow

If you hear the word *meditation*, you may think of an older man with a long beard, robe and no shoes. Well, it's time to change that image. The damaging effects of the loud, chaotic world are many, and the true purpose of meditation is to make your mind calm and peaceful and to decrease stress. When your mind is peaceful and quiet, you will be freer from worry, stress, anxiety, and fear.

Here are two meditation techniques that are easy to do:

1. Counting breaths

The first stage of meditation is to stop distractions and make your mind clear. This can be done by beginning with a simple breathing meditation.

You can start in any position you are comfortable with. Close your eyes and concentrate on your breathing. Breathe in through your nose and out through your nose. Breathe naturally, and don't try and control your breathing. Just concentrate on your nostrils. The sensation you feel in and out of your nostrils is where all your concentration is going to be. You will try to concentrate on that, excluding everything else.

Your mind at first will begin to wander. That's OK, because it is showing you how busy it always is. Just

> You're in a daily war fighting against disease, debt, emotional turmoil, weight gain, shrinking muscles, divorce and failed relationships. As a parent, you're fighting all of the enemies that would block your children's health and future.

slowly go back to concentrating on your breathing through your nostrils. As soon as a thought comes in, go back to concentrating on your breathing.

Next, you will begin counting your breaths. Breathe in through the nose and then out through the nose for the first count. Count up to five, and then start again at one. If you lose count, it's because you're not focusing. Don't get frustrated; just start over at one. Keep counting sets of five breaths for at least five minutes. Gradually work your way up to fifteen minutes per day. The more you do this, the easier it becomes and the more relaxed you will feel.

2. Natural breathing

Once you have mastered counting your breaths, it's time to begin the next level of meditation. This meditation is done the same way as the counting breaths, except that instead of counting, you just breathe naturally. Do not control it. Let your body do the breathing, realizing that it is happening without you thinking about it. If you have mastered counting your breaths, then you will have the focus as soon as something pops into your mind to refocus back on your breathing.

Starting each day with mental exercise like meditation will instill a new sense of passion and excitement in your life. More than anything, it helps you focus on what's important in life which will reduce your mental and emotional stress and make your day fun and exciting. One aspect of the human brain is that whatever it focuses on is almost always what it gets. You will ultimately attract what you focus on daily.

> The problem never truly is that there is not enough time; the problem is that there is not enough *time management*.

> The man who acquires the ability to take full possession of his own mind may take possession of anything else to which he is justly entitled.
> ~ Andrew Carnegie

> Everything you want is out there waiting for you to ask. Everything you want also wants you. But you have to take action to get it.
> ~ Jack Canfield, author, *Chicken Soup for the Soul*

The Maximized Life and Challenges

> So much time, so little to do.... Wait... Reverse that.
> ~ Gene Wilder as Willy Wonka

A Personal Note from Dr. Ben Lerner

What would it be like to have so much time on your hands that you don't know what to do—without being incarcerated or lost on a deserted island with no one to talk to but Wilson? Most people couldn't imagine that. We get up and go, go, go; and we usually get up before we've had the necessary amount of sleep to be mentally or physically well.

The really bizarre part about how busy we are is that our culture is suffering in most, if not all, of the important areas of life—family, health, finances, and fulfillment. They are in the worst shape they have ever been in! This, of course, begs the question, "What are we so busy doing?"

From the moment of your birth forward, you're allotted a very specific amount of time in your life. No matter what you believe, your days are numbered. If you live long enough, eventually you're going to die. Last time I checked, death was still affecting one out of every one of us. Therefore, all that ultimately matters while on earth is what you do with each one of the days that you have. Many aren't making the best choices for how limited those days really are.

In my life when I've been the busiest, I've never been the most successful. First of all, when I let rushing overtake me, I start making bad choices for my life. When I'm rushing to and fro, I start missing sleep, eating badly, letting my preferred exercise schedule slide, spending less time with my wife and kids, and shortening my peace management time. And those are just the obvious problems.

Even worse, as I look back to the times I've been the most rushed, I find that I operated through those times on autopilot. Moving toward that day of, "When I just past this one deadline," or "When I have this much money," or

MaximizedLivingMakeover.com

WAR PLAN
Download a To-Do List and War Plan pages. View a sample To-Do List and War Plan page from Dr. Ben Lerner.

> If you don't have a clear, safe path and strategy, life's going to hurt.

WINNING THE PEACE TRIATHLON

Write about your experiences and learn from the experiences of others.

Focused energy on an area of your life is present-time consciousness or "up time" (UT).

"As soon as this project gets completed," it's like I'm in a coma. Days, weeks, months, and even years can rush by.

You're just getting *through* time and rarely getting much *from* your time. You can spin like a hamster on a wheel with the belief in front of you that there's some kind of promised land-on-earth type of destination where you'll just stop and enjoy life—but never getting there! That's the opposite of maximized living!

During these times, you also make terrible choices. Being overworked, underrested, and negatively stressed badly affects your decision-making ability. Not only are you messing up your life by rushing through it, but also you further aggravate the situation by making wrong decisions.

Your life is now! If you're not experiencing joy and health *now* and you're not working on and investing in your joy and health for later, you're blowing it! Destination living is the proverbial way of missing your whole life and destroying everything that's important.

When life events rush in and knock you out of your yellow boxes, sit back down with your solid yellow box planner and create a plan for what you think would be the greatest year of your life. Cut off with a chainsaw many of the things that drain days and literally take the life out of what's really important. You have to be brutal. This won't be an easy task, because you won't want to cut them off or you wouldn't have put them there in the first place. But do barbaric surgery on them anyway. (This is one case where surgery is A-OK!)

After my first book, *Body By God,* landed on the *New York Times* bestsellers list, I had an opportunity to speak all over the world. As much as I loved doing it, reached many lives, and profited financially from it, it took too much time away from my family and my health. The bottom line was, it just didn't feel right. Rather than doing what many people do and just keep going, pushing, and traveling the world, I took a knife to it. I cut the amount of times annually that I'm available to speak from fifty down to fifteen. You know what? It's worked out great. I'm booked a year in advance, everyone's happy at home, and I've got "So much time, so little to do." Of course, I'm still very busy; but I'm busy with what's important!

What's important for your future is maximized living. The future is coming. You can either invest now and experience maximized living when the future arrives, or keep withdrawing from your mind, body, and emotions now and experience something much, much less. Either way, it's up to you.

Now it's time for you to dive into one of the thirty-day Maximized Living makeover challenges. Each challenge takes you deeper into the five essentials and gives you practical, easy-to-do daily steps to get you closer to your goals of maximized living.

If the concepts in this book are largely new to you, or if you recognize that you are overworked, overstressed, and out of shape, start with the Beginner Makeover Challenge for the next thirty days. Dr. Greg Loman's easy-to-follow and engaging entries give you bite-sized action steps to start enjoying the benefits of Maximized Living advantages from day one!

By the time you reach day 30, or if you are in fairly good shape and want more of a challenge, the Intermediate Makeover is the one for you. Go deeper in maximizing your strengths in all of the essentials—from GPS positioning to delving into your unique talent proposition—plus daily action steps on diet, exercise, nerve supply, and eliminating toxins. You can work the Intermediate Makeover Challenge once or go through it again and again until the positive, life-changing steps become lifelong healthy habits.

Finally, you can find Dr. Charles Major's Elite Makeover Challenge at the end of each day of the Intermediate Challenge. The two challenges can be done simultaneously, or the Elite Makeover Challenge can stand alone or follow the Intermediate Makeover Challenge. It takes you even further down the path of wellness and maximized living.

Turn the page and get ready to take the Maximized Living challenge. Whether you're a beginner, intermediate, or elite, start today. It doesn't matter so much where you are right now; it matters only that you get moving on a path toward a healthier life. Your true worth is not your current state, but your potential state.

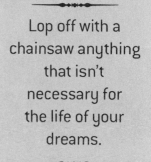

> Lop off with a chainsaw anything that isn't necessary for the life of your dreams.

> You're either growing or dying. So in order to keep the mission alive, plan daily and weekly growth.

MaximizedLivingMakeover.com

YOUR GPS FORM

Download a "GPS" form and view a sample one from Dr. Ben Lerner.

> To live to the fullest mentally, emotionally, spiritually, financially, and relationally, then we have to prepare our mental and emotional states.

Remember, you matter! Your family needs you, your friends need you, and the world around you needs your unique skills, talents, and capabilities. And you can serve them best by being the best you—the you that is experiencing maximized living!

TAKE A STEP FORWARD!

1. True Maximized Living encompasses and benefits all aspects of your life, and that includes your emotions, relationships, and the amount of peace you have. This is not just because the point of life is to enjoy it, it's also because lack of peace actually has impact on the duration of life. To learn more about the connection between peace and the incidence of heart disease and cancer, be sure to go to the reports on www.MaximizedLivingMakeover.com

2. Stress is not just a problem, it's an epidemic. Six of the top 10 medications sold today are being prescribed for depression and anxiety. You don't need less stress; you need more peace. Think about how to implement more peace in your life today!

3. You add peace to your life as you gain new perspectives. It's important to lean into the Five Steps for Improving Your Perspective on Life, which are:

   - Recognize your value
   - Discover your UTP: Unique Talent Proposition
   - Find a Higher Purpose
   - Create a Personal Value System
   - Dismiss Results and Reactions

   If you haven't already watched the in-depth video or written down your UTP, please do so now by getting something to write with and going to www.MaximizedLivingMakeover.com

4. Getting control of your time means getting control of your life. You don't stumble on a great life—you schedule it! At www.MaximizedLivingMakeover.com, you can download planning forms and learn to use them. If you're not sure what to write down, be sure to look at the sample pages.

5. You have nine lives—make them extraordinary by scheduling time for all of them and sticking to it!

6. Practice the Peace Triathlon. Write about your experiences and learn from the experiences of others at www. MaximizedLivingMakeover.com. While you are there, also view our recommendations for positive, inspiring, and empowering literature.

7. Keep going to the next section. Section the "30 Day Challenge" that is right for you!

By strengthening your mind and tending your heart (emotions), you prepare your will, fortify your resolve, and continue your journey to building peace.

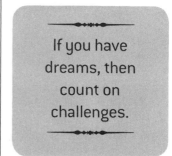

If you have dreams, then count on challenges.

PART TWO

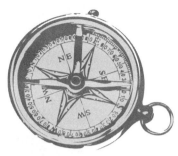

The Maximized Living
Makeover Challenges

Let's Get This Party Started!

Now that you have a good idea of what it means to live a maximized life, we can almost hear what you are thinking: *How on earth do I get there?* Don't panic. The point of opening your eyes to all of the ways you may *not* be experiencing maximized living is not to scare you, overwhelm you, or make you feel guilty. Not at all!

The entire reason for this book is to inspire you to make small changes every day that will set you on the path to the way of maximized living you truly want and deserve. And your family too! By adding and subtracting small things in your life each day, you can make a huge difference in the way you look, feel, and experience life.

In this last section of *Maximized Living Makeover* we, Dr. Lerner, Dr. Loman, and Dr. Majors, want to help you get started on a new way of living that will benefit you and your family for the rest of your lives. We have put together a series of three thirty-day Maximized Living Makeover challenges. The first one, written by Dr. Loman, is designed for the beginner—the average person who hasn't really considered a lot of these ideas before and who wants to begin a few baby steps at a time to develop a healthier lifestyle on the way to maximized living.

The Beginner Makeover Challenge touches on ways to de-stress, refresh, eat healthier, and move more. It offers simple action steps that everyone can accomplish and feel great about. It is divided into important life categories that focus on inspiration, exercise, stress management, nutrition, and time management. Every three days you will take action steps in one of these categories, then move to the next one. Each day of the challenge that you accomplish, we promise that you will feel better and be closer to your goal of maximized living.

The second challenge is the Intermediate Makeover Challenge of the Maximized Living Makeover, written by Dr. Lerner. It is designed for the person who already has a fitness plan, employs good eating habits and follows some of the steps outlined in the five essentials. The Intermediate Makeover Challenge takes the Beginner Makeover Challenge and adds more elements to it so that you can get even closer to your goal of true maximized living in every area of your life. It offers detailed time-management plans, eating plans, and exercise suggestions.

Finally, the Elite Makeover Challenge by Dr. Lerner and Dr. Majors is created for those who are already serious athletes and fitness buffs, those who want to improve their lives but who are already well toned. The elite people are ready to go further in maximizing their lifestyle and explore other areas they may need to strengthen. You'll find the Elite Makeover Challenge at the end of each Intermediate Makeover Challenge entry, so you can go even deeper if you choose.

All three Maximized Living Makeover challenges have been formulated to be easy to dive into—nothing scary or overwhelming—and were written with enough helpful suggestions to get you going. There are just enough days in the thirty-day makeovers to get you in the habit of making positive changes in your life. We predict that you will be so thrilled with the way you feel that you'll want to complete all of the challenges—and may log on to www.MaximizedLivingMakeover.com to ask for more!

So what are you waiting for? Dive in to the right makeover challenge for you, and get started on your way to Maximized Living.

BEGINNER MAKEOVER CHALLENGE

By

Dr. Greg Loman

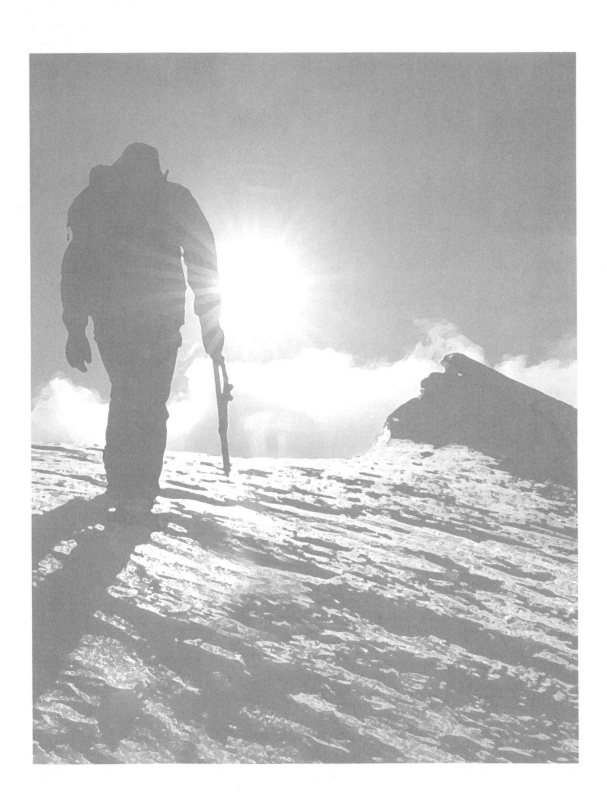

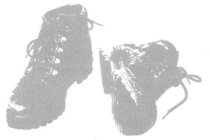

Day 1

INSPIRATION: Time for a New Life

Our whole lives we have been told we cannot do things. If you remember when you were a child, you were probably told no more than you were told yes. If you have children of your own, you know they ask, ask, ask. Children seem to have this unquenchable desire to explore everything and try anything. When I was young, I thought I could fly. I tried it once out of my tree fort. Boy, did that hurt.

My point is that children have no fear. They believe they can become anything, and when they get hurt, they try again. I'm not sure if it is the influence of adults that shuts down this willingness to be adventurous or bad results of children's experiments. Either way, the bottom line is that as adults we need to be as adventurous and willing to try new things as we were when we were children.

I remember a time when I was on vacation with my family on an island. I was in my boat working, and all I could hear was my father saying, about every sixty seconds or so, "Ki, stop jumping from that. You are going to hurt yourself." I decided to watch what was going on. My son, who was then only three years old, was jumping off a ledge more than twice his height. He would jump, run around, climb stairs to the ledge and jump again.

Once I saw what Ki was doing and saw that it was safe, I stopped what I was doing and went over to my young son. I got his attention and said, "Ki, do not let Poppy tell you that you can't do that. Never let anyone tell you that you cannot accomplish something."

That's something to remember as you begin the first challenge in Maximized Living. Getting started always seems like the hardest part. When you are on an island and it seems like you are the only one on that island, starting is 90 percent of the battle. I know the island of procrastination, uncertainty and fear is lonely. However, you are not alone. Many are there with you. The key is just to make the first move. The move does not even need to be a big one—just get moving, and you'll be on your way to Maximized Living.

Let me tell you a story to encourage you as you begin. Tyler is a young man in his early twenties who works for me. Tyler, like many of us, was raised in the typical American environment of plenty of TV, video games, and processed foods. His family did not gear their time around taking care of themselves with the Maximized Living principles and essentials in mind. In fact, there was minimal or no inspiration for Tyler to take care of his health. Tyler's family joined the rest of the 99 percent of American families who are not geared around maximizing life, health, and existence.

Due to this lifestyle, Tyler slowly gained weight. Over a decade, he gained a lot. His health started declining. He started sleeping poorly. His energy slowly dwindled. His diminished organ function started to affect his daily life. By the time he was in his early twenties and came to us, he had sixty more pounds than his body could handle, and back problems set in due to his weight. Ulcers and digestive problems developed. Headaches then followed. All of these problems developed by the time this young man was barely out of his teens.

Tyler decided to do something about his problem. I invited Tyler to join me and the other doctors I work with on our Wednesday morning run. That first Wednesday, Tyler did not show up. In fact, it took Tyler three more weeks before he finally showed up at our six o'clock in the morning run. That morning, I decided to ask Tyler what had happened the other times he missed.

He responded, "The first night before the run I started to set my alarm for 5:30 a.m., but I became fearful so I set it for my normal time of 6:30 a.m. The second week I set my alarm, and the alarm went off at 5:30 a.m. However, I did not want to get up and went back to bed. The third week I got up and actually was dressed before I bailed. I was embarrassed to run with everyone. Finally, the fourth time I was so mad that I pushed myself and showed up for the run."

When Tyler finally showed up for the run, I told him only to push himself to his own capacity—then to give an extra 10 percent. I told him not to try and compete with the other runners.

◪Note: While it may be hard for men who are reading this book, it is important to note that you are only competing against yourself. Lay your ego aside, and do your own personal best. Ego can be destructive and counterproductive. Lay it down!

Tyler listened and walked most of that first time. Six months later, he still walks some; however, he also jogs a portion of our exercise time.

Tyler's life is now changed forever. He started a corrective chiropractic program, exercises and changed the way he eats. The key to Tyler's story is that he began to change slowly. He found a place to start and, like most people, makes changes slowly. This approach is better than trying to climb Mount Everest today. Most will fail and never try again because it is too hard. Due to Tyler's commitment in the last six months, he no longer gets headaches. His back pain is gone, his digestion has improved tremendously and he sleeps more soundly. Oh, yeah, he smiles a lot more now too!

The greatest mistake you can make in your life is to quit before you start. In Tyler's case it was OK that he did not show up the first time. In fact, it was OK that he didn't show up the next couple of times. It was perfectly fine that Tyler showed up when it was right for him. The key was that he finally showed up.

It is OK to fail many times before you make something happen. Thomas Edison failed 1,000 times before he invented a functional light bulb. Actually, Edison did not fail at all; he merely found 999 ways *not* to make the light bulb.

Colonel Sanders, the developer of Kentucky Fried Chicken, at first could not give away his fried chicken recipe. He took it to hundreds of restaurants before one person said yes. He also did not start his first Kentucky Fried Chicken until he was in his sixties. Yet look at that fast-food chain today!

The Bottom Line for Day 1

It is never too late to get started in life, and it is never too late to succeed.

Action Step

Find a time and a place to read *Maximized Living Makeover* daily.

Day 2

INSPIRATION: The Maximized Living Financial Portfolio

When you want to accomplish something in life, having a powerful purpose for doing it is greater than the action you put into getting it done. For many people, the reason they choose to start a program like ours is to lose weight or look better. Most of the time, the reasons people start are health- or looks-related.

Those are fine reasons, but have you also thought about the financial gain as a motivating factor for wanting to embark on Maximized Living? OK, I know you are probably thinking, "How could spending money on this book, new walking shoes, and health food *save* me money?"

Would you believe me if I told you that if you properly follow this program, you will save hundreds of thousands of dollars, putting them right back in your wallet where they belong?

Let me explain. New statistics show that more than 60 percent of all bankruptcies are due to health-related problems. Not a day goes by in most cities in America that you do not see a television commercial that relates to bankruptcy. It is a crime that someone would work his or her whole life and save properly, only to watch (or worse, allow) a health problem to take all their money. Maybe you are thinking that most of these bankruptcies are tied to serious tragedies like automobile or industry accidents. That's simply not the case. In more than 80 percent of the bankruptcies filed because of health issues, the health issue at fault is chronic disease.

By taking the time to engage in the Maximized Living makeover, you are on your way to becoming healthier. Think of the instructors of this program as the greatest stockbrokers or hedge fund managers in your area.

Below are some of the multiple ways you will save and make money, if the Maximized Living plan is followed properly. If you save wisely, you could be a millionaire by the time you are sixty-five. Disclaimer: *Unless you waited until the age of sixty to start this program!*

Health Savings via the Maximized Living Makeover
1. Headaches: general—$20.00 per month over-the-counter medication = $240 per year.
2. Headaches: chronic—doctor visits, blood tests, MRIs, injections, neurologists, prescription narcotics. Out-of-pocket per year expenses = $1,000 to $3,000 per year.

3. Chronic pain: general—over-the-counter medication, doctor visits, x-rays, MRIs, injections, other medical tests, surgery = $1,000 to $3,000 (conservative estimate) per year. If surgery needed, up to $100,000.

4. Adult-onset diabetes: medications (Insulin)—$100 to $400 per month, depending on the severity; hospital visits—$3,000 to $25,000 per stay. Research shows that each new diabetic patient increases the income of an endocrinologist $250,000 over the lifetime of the patient.

*** Chronic disease can cost between $1,000 and $25,000 per year on average. This includes doctor visits, medications, surgeries, missed work hours, and loss of productivity if you own your own business.***

The Bottom Line for Day 2

Maximized Living Makeover = becoming a health millionaire.

Action Step

Look at your schedule for the next thirty-three days and identify the areas or situation that may interfere with your daily reading. If you find days that are too packed with events, alter your schedule to allow time to get your reading in. Do not let anything get in your way. Put your daily reading in the schedule and guard that time like you work at Fort Knox!

Day 3

INSPIRATION: Let's Not Kill Ourselves

One of the most destructive principles anyone could live by is the all-or-none principle. All too often I see people give up or never start because they cannot follow through with a certain task or give an activity 100 percent.

I call it the "Success 101" factor. As a life coach and health mentor, when I ask people questions, I typically get what you would call the "success" answer from people rather than the answer that is based in reality. It is almost as if the person is thinking, "I know what I should be saying to the doctor so I will say that because that is the successful answer."

As important as it is to strive to be the most productive person you can be and to be a committed person to maximizing your life, thinking that you can experience Maximized Living from day 1 (or day 3, in this case) is unrealistic. Wanting complete change *now* is many times the quickest way to depression and a setup for complete failure.

For example, if I asked the question, "If you were to die tomorrow, what would you have wanted your life to look like today?" here is the Success 101 answer:

1. I would like to have had $5 million.
2. I would like to have exercised daily for two hours—and been able to run a 5K in five-minute miles.
3. I would like to have had 4.2 percent body fat.
4. I would have traveled the world, visiting twenty-five countries.
5. I would have eaten only organic food.
6. I would have had a time-managed life where I properly utilized every minute of the day.
7. I would have had total love from family.
8. I would have owned my own business that developed a foundation for suffering children.

If you are like many, as you sat down and started to dream of how you would want your life to look like in the end, your imagination would have come up with amazing things—but many of them would not look like your real life today. The hard part is to create a list like the one above and make it a reality. Live it out.

I would never want to inhibit your dreams or stop you from believing you can accomplish the life of your dreams. But I want you to see that looking at the dream list can be overwhelming for most. This is especially true if you are not doing the things right in your life today that would get you anywhere near achieving that list.

Many would look at that list and stop before they started. That's the all-or-none principle. Many people want it all right now, but they are not willing to start taking the steps needed to get there one day at a time. As a beginner at mastering your life, you must be OK with taking baby steps.

⚡Note: It is important to note that in this thirty-day Beginner Makeover Challenge, you may only begin to master one or two areas of the Five Essentials needed in your life.

Consider this recent example of a woman who participated in one of the Extreme Makeover God's Way, a health make over for Christians we offer in our Maximized Living Centers:

Linda is a middle-aged woman who—due to some changes in her circumstances and finances—needed to take on multiple jobs to make ends meet. In the past, she had led a simpler life. Now, Linda found herself time crunched and stressed. As this added stress was put upon her life, she began to feel pressured. The additional work hours in her schedule caused her not to have as much time for sleep. This resulted in her becoming tired. Her exhaustion wore down her normally energetic personality.

Because Linda now had fewer hours of free time, her eating habits changed. She had less time to prepare food and began making poor food choices and developing bad habits. The additional jobs also interfered with Linda's exercise habits. Linda used to take time to walk multiple times per week. This activity began to slowly dwindle down to eventually nothing. She quit walking because she did not have time.

By this point in her life, Linda had become unhappy and stressed. How did it happen? When did it happen? Linda was formerly a happy, positive, energetic person. Now she was out of shape, out of sleep, and her life was basically out of control.

Linda began to realize that she needed a change, but she did not know how to change. Once she began to explore her situation, she tried to make adjustments. However, when you are stuck in the middle of a tornado, it is hard to see what's really happening around you. "It's too overwhelming," she thought.

There were many layers to Linda's problem:
1. Poor sleeping habits
2. Poor eating habits
3. Poor time management
4. No exercise

She then decided to sign up for the makeover in our office. Just four short weeks later, Linda's life was changed forever. We could see it in her face. Her attitude changed, her energy began to come back, and happiness set in. As I spoke to Linda about her transformation, I was sure she would tell me that she had employed all of our suggested strategies and transformed every area of her life. I was positive that such a dramatic change could only have occurred if Linda had become one of those miracle stories. I just knew she had joined a gym, developed a complete time-management schedule, and switched to shopping only at organic grocery stores.

I was wrong.

As I interviewed her for this book, Linda told me that in the four weeks she had only changed one thing. One! She had looked at her schedule and switched when she worked. She moved a few shifts to the night shift where she was able to multitask and get some home responsibilities accomplished while she was at work.

1. I asked rather incredulously, "Is that all you changed? I'll admit I am surprised."
2. "I could not believe it, Dr. Loman," Linda said with a smile I will never forget. "One little thing changed, and it felt like a car was taken off my shoulders."
3. Now that Linda has changed that one issue in her life, she can move on to achieve bigger goals. She will be able to move into the Intermediate and Elite Makeover Challenges if she chooses.

The Bottom Line for Day 3:

Be OK with moving forward at your own pace. Do not compare your growth in life to people around you. Put a microscope on your life and your situation, and then move toward your goal.

This can be a hard one for women. Most women put everyone else in the family first and themselves last, but it's OK to remember the classic line: "If momma ain't happy, nobody's happy." It is OK, in fact, it is *necessary*, to take care of yourself!

Action Step

Pick five realistic goals or outcomes to achieve by the time you reach day 30.

1. _____

2. _____

3. _____

4. _____

5. _____

Day 4

EXERCISE: You Can Have Fun Now...

We spent the first three days of the Beginner Makeover Challenge giving you inspiration for the journey, and hopefully getting you excited about the great changes you are going to make—one day at a time—during these first steps toward maximized living.

Now for the next three days we will begin to slowly engage in exercise. Exercise is a tricky subject, and it almost always elicits a gut response for the beginner—the overworked and out of shape—of depression and embarrassment. If I had you close your eyes and then asked you to describe the picture you get when you think of exercise, what would that look like? For many, the first description starts with negative emotions.

Beginners tend to immediately picture this gym full of bodybuilders and women who look like they do sit-ups in their sleep. Walking into a gym when you are out of shape can be a nightmare. Going to the dentist to have teeth extracted would be less painful than showing off your body in front of the more perfect ones all around you. The time for gyms may come later, but for now, let's find different, easier forms of exercise that will help you begin to move your body without any embarrassment at all. The point is not where you get your body moving, the point is just to get it moving!

The Bottom Line for Day 4

Start exercising slowly and in a setting where you won't feel embarrassed. Most importantly , pick an activity you like to do! (Personally, I do not like running so I bicycle. I actually enjoy seeing land rush by under my feet at twenty-five miles per hours.)

Action Step

Pick three activities you enjoy. (Exercise)

1. _____

2. _____

3. _____

Day 5

EXERCISE: Just Get Moving

The alarm goes off. It is six o'clock in the morning and you feel like you've been hit by a truck. Have you ever been there? Maybe even this morning? Maybe you think you are the only one who feels this way, but many of us do not like getting up early. Most of us have that moment before the feet hit the floor when confusion and delusion make our heads spin. Our eyes cannot focus, we feel weak, and on and on.

The most amazing thing happens in the next few minutes, doesn't it? Within a few minutes of waking, everything gradually becomes clear. It is as if someone turned on the light bulb. Thank God for that light bulb because some days you wonder if you will ever get moving.

Have you ever had that same feeling when you watched TV for a long period of time? Think back to a time when you watched TV all day. If you got up to go to the refrigerator, you probably almost thought, "Maybe I am sick, or I did not get enough sleep last night," because of the lethargic feeling. This also happens if you have ever traveled for long distances in a car. When you finally climb out of the car, you almost feel groggy, as if you need a nap. All of these situations have nothing to do with tiredness, sickness, or even laziness.

Physiologically, the body goes into a state of inactivity when it lacks movement. It is a lot like your computer. When you do not use a computer for a certain period of time, it goes into sleep mode. (Sometimes that drives me up a wall trying to get the computer to start moving again.)

Your body is the same way. It really was not created to sit. It was created to move. You might be thinking, "Not mine!" But I can assure you that yes, even yours, was created to move. Every one of the situations described above illustrates the point. In each of those situations, once you start moving, the lethargy dissipates and suddenly (or sometimes gradually) you come alive.

Today's plan is to recognize that your body wants to move, and now is the time you will start to move it more. Maybe we can substitute the phrase "move more" for the nasty word *exercise*. As a beginning mover, here is a simple tip to help you start moving your body. Pick three places where you can walk farther to get to your destination, for example:

1. Park in the parking spot at the mall that is farthest from the door.
2. Park in the spot at work that is farthest from the door.
3. Use stairs instead of the elevator.

The Bottom Line for Day 5

Begin to move more.

Action Step

Pick three destinations to walk farther.

1. _____

2. _____

3. _____

Day 6

EXERCISE:
"The Sun Is Always Shining; Only Clouds Get in the Way"

This is one of my favorite sayings because it can describe many aspects of our lives. It basically says that even with all of the troubles in life, things are actually OK if you choose to see them that way. Believe it or not, you can believe that there is sun behind the clouds, but also you can move the clouds out of the way! It is up to you.

At times, our lives seem gloomy. We have a bad day, our boss yells at us, our car breaks down, our dog dies, or maybe nothing particularly bad has happened at all. It is just a bad day. It does not matter who you are; everyone has bad days. You may think, "Well, look at her. She is beautiful; she never has a bad day," or, "He is a millionaire. If I had the money he has, I would never have a bad day."

Go and talk to those people. They have just as many bad days as you do. Sometimes it's easy to feel that we are the only ones having bad days. Rest assured, you are not by yourself. The difference between the happy and the unhappy is that the happy decided to *move the clouds out of the way*.

One of the best ways to move the clouds out of the way is to get your body moving. (Remember, we're not using the *exercise* word.) Today, or in the next few days when you are having a bad one, you still have the capacity to move. And when you do, you'll start moving those clouds right out of your line of sight. Pretty soon, the sun will be shining again.

If you are having a fight with your spouse or someone close to you, get in the car and travel to the beach, a lake, or your favorite park and move that body. If you can't go anywhere, just step outside and go for a brisk walk or jog around the block. As the oxygen enters your lungs and your brain releases the chemicals that exercise produces, you will be amazed at how calm, relaxed, and, yes, even happy you begin to feel—even on a bad day!

The Bottom Line for Day 6

Move the clouds out of the way.

Action Step

Make a choice to move the clouds out of the way. Go ahead and try it. It is amazing to begin to recognize that you can change the way you feel about the day. Today, pick three places you are going to use in the moments when you need to move the clouds out of the way. When frustration comes, you feel irritated, or you just begin to feel lethargic, get up and move. Walk as briskly as you can for fifteen minutes. Then watch the magic happen.

My Move-the-Clouds-Out-of-the-Way Place(s)

1. _____

2. _____

3. _____

Day 7

STRESS MANAGEMENT: Take Time for Yourself

When financial experts advise people on how to manage their money, one of the first things they say is that you should always pay yourself first. What they mean is that you should take a percentage of your paycheck right off the top and save it for yourself before it is all spent on bills and obligations. The same is true for your time. You have to slow down and pay yourself in time if you want to be happy and healthy.

It is a well-known fact that stress is, if not the number-one cause of disease, definitely one of the top three. As much as this book is about health, many of our illustrations are directed toward stress-related issues. If stress affects our health so much, what about our happiness? Show me a happy person, and I will show you a healthy person with a relatively low level of stress. It all goes hand in hand in Maximized Living.

On day 3, I used the old saying, "If momma ain't happy, nobody is happy." We know this to be true, but what about daddy, the children, and the dog? Even though our nation has become self-centered and selfish in many ways, I also believe that all too often our lives are about chores, commitments, and obligations that do not feed or care for our bodies, our hearts, our minds, or our spirits.

When was the last time you took time for yourself? If your life is not filled with energy and happiness, how can you give to others? Even though my responsibilities as a father, husband, life coach, and multiple business owner are great and could consume every waking moment of my life, I still need to make time for myself.

In my house we call it "Daddy's time." Ask anyone in my family when Daddy's time is, and they will tell you it is Friday afternoon. When I am in town, Friday afternoon is my time for myself. Many times my wife asks me, "What are you going to do on Daddy's day?" I respond, "I don't know."

Really, many Fridays I don't know. Sometimes I just drive. The point is that once a week I take a few hours to de-stress. I can have fun, do nothing, have no responsibility... I just get to enjoy life. Many weeks I have more that that one time on Friday afternoon. The point is that with all my responsibilities, I have to schedule it in and protect that time slot carefully. No one can touch it. It is necessary to keep me happy and healthy.

> Most folks are about as happy as they make up their minds to be.
> ~ Abraham Lincoln

When was the last time you took time to let your hair down, dumped the load of stress, and made yourself happy? When was the last time you did something you really enjoy? Or have you forgotten what actually makes you happy?

The Bottom Line for Day 7

Pay some of your time to yourself. Schedule it in and stick to it.

Action Step

Write down three things that make you happy and do them.

1. _____

2. _____

3. _____

Day 8

STRESS MANAGEMENT: **If Momma or Daddy Ain't Happy...**

Remember when life was simple? Remember when people actually knew their neighbors? Remember when you would drive to the grocery store, and no one irritated you as you drove down the road? (You know, that crazy cell phone that sits on the passenger seat next to you. Oh, yours is always in your hand...That explains a lot about the way you drive.)

Believe it or not, all the "time-saving" technologies that have entered our lives have created stress like you cannot imagine. It's not feasible to give up technology, but we must learn to adapt so that technology doesn't push us over the edge. There are times you probably wish you lived on a farm, raised your own food, washed your clothes with the old-fashioned clothes thingy, and never saw another person until you made it to heaven. Believe me, we understand. Even as Maximized Living practitioners, we feel the same way many times each month.

Since moving to the woods is most likely not a viable answer for most of us, we need to address new technology and figure out what we can do to relieve this additional stress load. Here's a thought: how about an old-fashioned nap?

A nap? Aren't naps for wimps? Real men and women with time-crunched schedules can't possibly fit in a nap, right? I can hear you now, saying, "You do not understand. I have three children, a dog, and a home business. I don't have time for a nap."

The fact is, no one just has extra time lying around (pardon the pun). But you do have time—if you schedule it. And if you do, I promise, if you pencil in time for a nap, you are not a wimp. (And the benefits we believe you'll receive are so tremendous that you won't care if anyone thinks you're a wimp!) A nap will give you a refreshed outlook on life and restore your energy. This reduces your stress.

A key point to address is how long the nap is. The nap we are recommending is not the type where you undress, set the alarm for two hours later, and crawl in bed. The nap we are talking about is a power nap. It should only take ten to twenty minutes. Even with three children at home or work to do—whatever your unique situation—there is a way to make a power nap work for you. Here are a few examples:

1. If you are at work, take your fifteen-minute break in the afternoon. Buy a five-dollar alarm clock (and travel pillow, if you like), and bring it with you to work. At break time, find a quiet, dark place and turn off the lights. Lie on the floor and power nap.

2. At home, find a favorite movie for the children, lock yourself in your room, and set your alarm for ten minutes. Let the kids know they are not to bother you dur-

ing that short time unless someone is bleeding or there is a fire. If your child is an infant, take the advice of moms everywhere and nap while the baby is napping.

3. If you work and don't have a break scheduled, let your boss know that if you are refreshed by a short nap or rest period, you will produce better work. (Then, get ready to prove it.)

Obviously, these examples will not apply to every situation. But we believe that if you get creative, you can find a short period in most of your days to give yourself a much-needed "time out" to refresh yourself for the hours ahead. Try it. You'll be amazed at how much better you feel, and you will have taken another step toward your goal of maximized living.

The Bottom Line for Day 8
Small naps can provide great stress relief.

Action Step
Start taking short naps at work and at home.

Day 9

STRESS MANAGEMENT: Sticky Notes
Congratulations! You are well into your second week of the Maximized Living Beginners Makeover Challenge. Think about it: in eight days, the only things we have really worked on are inspiring you, getting you to move a little bit, and helping you to reduce stress by loving on yourself a little. See? It really is not that hard to work toward a maximized way of life, right?

For me one of the hardest issues I have faced in life is that my brain forgets everything.

My wife thinks things go in one ear and out the other. In fact, she has said that to me many times. To tell you the whole truth, I am willing to argue that most things do not even make it to the first ear. Never mind through my brain.

As easy as some of the tasks in this makeover challenge are, remembering them and getting into a habit—a routine—of doing them could be the hardest part of the thirty-day Maximized Living Makeover challenge. In fact, I would be willing to argue that most of your stress will come from trying to remember all of the changes you are supposed to be making. Memory management is truly one of the quickest ways to have this program fail for you.

Today, we will help you overcome that obstacle so that you can stick to your goals and keep on keepin' on. Day 9 is about one thing: sticky notes.

Sticky notes? What's the big deal about sticky notes? Let me tell you. Writing things down on sticky notes will actually reduce your stress tremendously. You can only keep a limited amount of information stored in the part of your brain responsible for instant recall. If sticky notes can be your instant-recall helpers, you don't have to feel like your brain is on overload. And you are less likely to forget the important details of life—like a meeting with your boss or the gallon of milk your wife told you to bring home.

When my wife first met me, I never forgot a single thing. Did I have a super brain back then? No. Have I lost my memory function since then? Not much (at least, I hope). I will admit that when someone entered my condo back then they would be faced with sticky notes everywhere—probably twenty at a time stuck to furniture, mirrors, the back of the front door and, of course, on my nightstand. They were my personal memory keepers.

Due to HGTV and my wife's desire for a neat, nice-looking home, which she says reduces *her* stress level, I am no longer allowed to leave sticky notes everywhere. This is also why I forget so many more things. My wife removed the one thing that helped my forgetful brain. So I adapted. Now, my sticky notes go in my belt.

The Bottom Line for Day 9

Get life's little details down on sticky notes to help you remember things and cut down on stress.

Action Step

Go to the store and buy sticky notes. Here are some ideas of where they might come in handy to help keep you organized and on the right track:

1. Put them on your dashboard in your car.
2. Stick them to the mirror where you brush your teeth.
3. Place them on your desk.
4. Take out your clothes the night before and place a note on your clothes.

Day 10

NUTRITION: Fuel for the Car

The theme for the next three days is shopping and eating out. Now don't get panicky. I will not be taking away your fried chicken, ice cream, or martinis. Why wouldn't I ask you to give up what you know is bad for you? Because the biggest reason most diets do not work is that you will naturally want to rebel when someone aggressively tells you what you have to do. And that's how many diets, weight-loss programs, and seminars go. A rambunctious, overly aggressive lecturer asks you to instantly give up your regular, comfortable eating habits and move immediately to the ever-so-painful, tofu-vegetables-water-and-gravel diet. For 90 percent of Americans, this is simply too hard. (Just in case you were wondering, the tofu-and-water diet is the basis of the Maximized Living Elite Makeover Challenge. Ha! Just kidding!)

Seriously, though, while we do need to start eating the right foods, it is just as important to make changes slowly so that you can adjust without feeling deprived and depressed. You can build up over months, even years, eventually becoming a healthier eater.

That being said, the sooner you make changes, the better you will begin to feel. One of the greatest reasons people experience diminished energy levels is that their "car" (body) has the nutritional equivalent of bad gas in it. For automobiles, the best way to fix a tank of bad gas is to empty the tank and only put good gas back in it. This is exactly the right answer for your body too. We need to start slowly adding good, healthy food to our already-established eating habits that we have been accustomed to for years.

Understand this clearly: this is not about taking anything away. Eat like you usually do. Just make it your goal to add a couple of healthy foods to your menu today (and every day from this day forward). Soon, you will find that the way you feel after eating healthy foods will prompt you to want more of them, eventually "weaning" you away from some of your bad habits without you even noticing!

The Bottom Line for Day 10

Good, healthy foods can be added to your menu each day without subtracting what you usually eat.

Action Step

Add one or two good, healthy foods to your diet today and every day from here forward. On your next shopping trip, plan to choose several items that you like that are healthy and add them to your shopping cart. You can find good choices in the health food section of traditional grocery stores, if you can't head to a local health food or organic market. Here are a few suggestions to get you started:

1. For breakfast, add a piece of fruit or a granola bar (but not the standard, sugar-filled, processed grocery store kind. Read labels and choose the truly healthy selection.)
2. A mid-morning snack could be nuts, fruit, an energy shake or smoothie.
3. For lunch, add a salad, vegetable, or piece of lean beef or chicken.
4. For an afternoon snack, see mid-morning snack.
5. At dinnertime, add a salad, vegetables, or healthy bread.

Day 11

NUTRITION: Take Little Steps

Recently, I was interviewing Linda, the patient who had graduated from our Extreme Makeover God's Way program that we mentioned in an earlier story. She made some big changes in her life by taking small steps. Now Linda leads a busy life, and many times she misses meals, as you likely do. One day, she came into the office very excited, and when I asked her why she seemed so thrilled, she replied, "Last week I was in a gas station and was in line to purchase a soda and a Danish. As I stood there, I decided to put the Danish back and exchange it for an apple."

This may not seem like a very big deal; however, a move like this means Linda is on her way—simply by taking small steps—to a healthier and happier body. Imagine what your body is saying when you take a bad item and exchange it for a good, healthy item. What do you think it says? Let me tell you. It is saying, "I love you!"

Now I promised that if you eat junk food or at fast-food restaurants, I was not going to ask you to stop. And I'm not. But I am asking that if you choose to grab a junk food snack, make some good food choices too. Have your chocolate chip cookies, but see if you can get ones that are made from whole grain flour, with molasses or honey instead of processed white flour and sugar. Or eat the chocolate chip cookies, but have a small glass of organic milk with them instead of that sugar-laden cola or chemical-filled diet soda. At a fast-food restaurant, choose the smallest value meal instead of upsizing it, or order water rather than that 32-ounce soda.

The Bottom Line for Day 11

Take small steps to create big changes.

Action Step

Exchange an unhealthy piece of food or snack for something healthy, especially if you are purchasing food at a gas station or fast-food restaurant. Yes, you can still have your soda or icee. Just exchange something else that is bad for something good.

Day 12

NUTRITION: Shop in the Horseshoe

Have you heard the joke about the young girl who asked her mom at Thanksgiving dinner why she cut the ends off of the ham before she put it in the pan to bake? Her mother responded, "I don't know. I always watched my mother, your grandmother, do it. So that's why I do it. Let's ask her why." So the mother asks the grandmother why the ends are cut off the ham, and the grandmother says, "I do not know. I always watched my mother do it that way, so let's ask her." So they asked the great-grandmother the same question, and she responded, "My pan was too small, so I cut the ends off so it would fit."

My point here is that we tend to do things in life just because our parents did them, without any regard to the reason why. We rarely even question where our habits came from or why we do things the way we do them. Shopping is one of those habits. When I was little, I remember the first place we would go in the grocery store is the cereal aisle. That was aisle 6 in our grocery store. Do not ask me how I remember that. Maybe I wrote it down on a sticky note when I was eleven.

But the cereal aisle, usually located in the middle of the store, isn't the healthiest place to be. Let me teach you a new way to shop at the grocery store. It will feel different than your usual habit, but if you begin to form a new habit of shopping this way, you'll find healthy eating easier—I promise! It may not be how your mother did it, but if you make a healthy change, it will be the way your kids do it.

We call it "shopping in the horseshoe." And it goes like this: the next time you enter the grocery store, make sure the first half of your shopping trip takes place around the complete outside perimeter of the store. If you think of the layout of most grocery stores, around the perimeter you will find the dairy items, produce section, and fresh meats. Things like cheeses, eggs, milk, meats, fruits, and vegetables are all on the outside—not the inside aisles of a grocery store.

Shopping in the horseshoe fills your cart with the live foods. The aisles in the middle have all the "dead" or preservative-filled foods. The first time you try this, it might feel difficult, but do it anyway. Go directly to the outside and shop there first. If you go directly to the middle aisles, you are far more likely to fill up your cart with unhealthy items and not have enough money left for the healthy choices around the perimeter!

The Bottom Line for Day 12

Shopping in the horseshoe fills your shopping cart with healthy, live foods.

Action Step

Shop the horseshoe at the grocery store.

Day 13

TIME MANAGEMENT: Finding Time

As we wrap up the second week of the Beginner Makeover Challenge, we have already taken many action steps to improve your life. Hopefully, you have carved out time for yourself, refreshed yourself with a few power naps, de-stressed by keeping details on sticky notes, gotten your body moving, and shopped the horseshoe for healthy foods. Congratulations! I know you are feeling better about yourself through these positive changes already.

For the next three days, we will focus on finding time. There are only twenty-four precious hours in each day, and every one of them needs to be spent living life to the max! We will find time by cutting activities out of the schedule, rescheduling other activities, or becoming more time-efficient in some areas. All you need to do to find extra time is to pinpoint one of these areas and make the necessary adjustment.

Sounds easy, doesn't it? But we all know that it's easier said than done. Time is the most elusive, confusing and most talked about stress factor on the planet. Being a doctor who gives recommendations for change on a daily basis, I hear the panicked words, "But I do not have time!" more times a day than I take breaths!

Can you imagine if we could purchase time? Wow, would that be expensive! And even if we could purchase more time, it would be like medical care, more expensive than we could ever afford. Instead of imagining unlikely scenarios (and wasting time in the process), let's get started uncovering the hidden time you didn't even know you had. When you apply the principles of the next three days, I promise you will have more time than you could imagine.

I believe the biggest issue with our overscheduled lives is the illusion that they are completely out of control. Not true! Your time—every minute of it—is completely under your control. You just have to take control of it. If you don't, it is amazing how just one additional issue, task, or appointment in an overscheduled life can throw an otherwise sane person totally over the edge. On the flip side, if you identify and get rid of the issues, tasks, or appointments that are throwing everything else off, you will feel like a ton of weight has just rolled off your shoulders.

The Bottom Line for Day 13

Your schedule may be out of control, but it is not out of your control. Take charge of your schedule and eliminate the time eaters that are putting you over the edge.

Action Step

At the end of the day today, do not turn on the TV. Tonight, take time by yourself or with your partner to find that one thing in your life (or a few things) that take time you should not spend. Get rid of those time eaters or reduce the time given to them. Here are a few examples:

1. Turn off the TV.
2. Spend less time on personal grooming.
3. Turn off the cell phone.
4. Cut down or eliminate socializing nightly.
5. Trim the amount of time spent shopping or window shopping.
6. Cut down on the number of sports activities weekly.
7. Cut down on the number of activities your children are involved in. Save time to be parents and be a family. Kids do not need fourteen activities per week to be well rounded. What they need most is to be parented.

Day 14

TIME MANAGEMENT: Reschedule

OK, remember the ham joke from day 12? The one about the family who kept cutting the ends off their hams simply because three generations ago a pan was too small? Many times we find ourselves locked into the same old patterns like that family, living the same way we always have. That doesn't work well when it comes to our schedules. If we never make changes, we start moving on automatic pilot, never evaluating whether a certain chore or task could be accomplished more effectively at a different point in our week.

For example, if you run to the grocery store to get food for dinner every day after work, you spend much more time on that errand than if you could move it to early on a weekday morning, late at night, or early on Saturday morning when the traffic is lighter and the crowds in the store are down. Another example could be housework. If you are used to giving up every Sunday afternoon and evening to washing, drying, and folding the many loads of laundry that have accumulated during the week, why not reevaluate and put one load in the washer and dryer each night, folding it and starting the next load the following morning? Just by putting a fresh spin on an old schedule, you may free up extra time for yourself.

As mentioned before, extra time means a less crowded schedule. And a less crowded schedule equals less stress on our bodies, minds, and spirits. So how do you spell relief?

R-E-S-C-H-E-D-U-L-E

The Bottom Line for Day 14

It's important to reevaluate our schedules on a regular basis and move chores and tasks to different times and days of the week to be more efficient.

Action Step

Find that one task, chore, or event that can be put into a different point in your week. Then try it in the new time slot. If it makes your day less hectic, lowers your stress, and/or takes less time, then keep it in the new time slot. If it doesn't, try it somewhere else. Here are a few suggestions:

1. Record your favorite show and watch it later.
2. Make the children's lunches (or your own) the night before, rather than on school and work mornings.
3. Change the time of day or day of the week that you grocery shop.

Day 15

TIME MANAGEMENT: Become More Efficient

I want to revisit the idea that time is the most talked about issue and stress-related problem on the planet. The reason for revisiting this is also to clarify again that *we* tend to cause this stress. Yes, we do it to ourselves. The good news is that since we made the problem, we also have the power to fix it ourselves.

The reason our world becomes so rocked and so stressed is partly caused by our lack of efficiency in different situations. We allow the world, our jobs, or other circumstances to dictate when we accomplish certain tasks.

⚡Note: The Beginner Makeover Challenge is just an overview and simple action steps that illustrate basic principles. We will get into more precise scheduling in the Maximized Living Intermediate Makeover Challenge.

Many times it is not the task or my work week that is overbearing; it is the interruptions. Having two children, ages four and six, causes me to feel like I have a couple of walking anchors tied to my feet during times when I am supposed to be accomplishing specific tasks. In fact, I have been interrupted writing the last few pages of this challenge!

The way you make time more efficient and effective is to identify tasks in your life where you are always interrupted. Imagine how quickly you could get something accomplished if...

1. The cell phone did not ring
2. A child did not walk into the room
3. A friend did not stop by
4. Your favorite show did not come on
5. Coworkers did not enter into the room

It's time to stop the interruptions—or at least cut down on them as much as possible. If you work at home, this may mean hiring a teen to help with the kids or the housework. It may mean grabbing the laptop and heading to a quiet restaurant or park for a few hours. It may mean deciding to check e-mail only at certain times once or twice a day instead of checking, deleting, and answering e-mails every few minutes. Finally (and perhaps this is the biggest interruption for many of us), it may mean turning off the cell phone during specific tasks. By cutting down or eliminating interruptions altogether, you can focus on the task at hand and get it done much more efficiently—saving you time and reducing your stress.

The Bottom Line for Day 15

You can save time and relieve stress by eliminating interruptions and focusing more efficiently on the tasks you must complete.

Action Step

Find the task or activity that is most interrupted in your life and stop the interruption. You will get that task accomplished in half the time—or less! (Really, we mean it. Turn off the cell phone.)

Day 16

INSPIRATION: Find Something You Love

Remember when you were a kid and you didn't think that you ever needed to sleep? You did not need an alarm clock, the sun, or your mommy to wake you up. In fact, if you had it your way, you would not go to sleep at night at all. Come on, you remember those days. I know it was a long time ago, but surely you can remember how nice it was to have all that energy. Where did it go?

I know you are thinking, "But I am grown now. I have responsibilities." I get it. I have responsibilities too and less energy to tackle them all, it seems, than when I was a boy. Welcome to adulthood.

One of the reasons life was great back then is that you had something to look forward to. You loved something. You anticipated the fun you would have. Two years ago at Christmas, my wife and I bought our son a battery-operated Cadillac Escalade. Boy, he thought he was in heaven. He spent every waking hour of the next month in the driveway, driving in circles. Yep, he was a speed demon at five miles per hour!

Do you have something you love with the same passion you felt as a kid? We don't have to get too serious here. Of course, you love your kids, your spouse, your family and close friends, and certainly you want to save the planet and feel passionately about that. But I'm talking about personal passion for something that you just love.

Seriously, when was the last time you did something fun or had something to look forward to? It is time to have some fun in life—even right smack dab in the middle of all your responsibilities.

Maybe you think you do not deserve to have fun. Maybe you were raised to be serious and accomplish great things in life. I understand where you are coming from, but you need to recharge with some fun in order to accomplish the serious tasks in life. Even overachievers like us need to make time for fun. I know you're thinking, "But you're already asking me to take time for myself each week and to build in power naps. You mean I have to find time for fun too?" My answer is, "Absolutely, yes!"

Laughter is a huge stress reliever. Taking pleasure in something makes life more exciting and makes obligations seem less difficult. Fun is, well, fun! Enough is enough! Go have some fun.

The Bottom Line for Day 16

Everyone needs to reignite the same sense of anticipation and excitement they felt as a child. Build some activities that are pure fun into your schedule.

Action Step

Find something you love to do, whether it is visiting a zoo or taking piano lessons. It does not need to be expensive or too time consuming. Just have some FUN.

Day 17

INSPIRATION: It's OK to Enjoy Life

Now that you have found something you love to do, make sure that you give yourself permission to stick with it. Make sure that you have found something that excites you. In fact, you should be so thrilled about this fun that you are having that it should make it difficult to get to sleep at night. (OK, so maybe that's a bit of an exaggeration.) The point here it to try to recapture some of the feeling you used to get as a kid when your parents told you that the next day you were going to Disney World, Sea World, or any other theme park. Try to rekindle that kind of thrill and anticipation over the fun activity you have chosen. If it's just ho-hum, pick another way to have fun!

Now that you have something to look forward to, make sure you actually get to enjoy it. Give yourself the time to do it, and give yourself permission to let your hair down and go with it. Fully immerse yourself in your times of fun. Don't make the mistake of spending your fun time on the cell phone, texting, on e-mail, or even just thinking about all the work you have waiting for you. And don't pencil in fun one week, then forget to make time for it for another two. Nothing is worse than finding something you love and, before you know it, allowing weeks to go by without doing it.

Pencil your fun times into your planner, your Blackberry, your PDA, your wall calendar, or my personal favorite from day 9—the sticky notes! In whatever way you choose, write it down. Make sure fun is put into your schedule. When you put it into your schedule, do not let anyone or any situation interfere with it. You need it, you deserve it, and—like we said in day 7—you can take time for yourself. It's OK. In fact, it's necessary for you to laugh, love, and live better. So don't feel guilty about taking some fun time. Today is the day to find something you love and take the time to experience it.

When you engage in activities that you enjoy, this releases certain chemicals in your brain that actually cause your body to function better through your nerve system. Fun not only brings joy, but also it brings better health through brain and nerve function.

> Most of us spend our lives as if we have another one in the bank.
> ~ Ben Erwin

The Bottom Line for Day 17

Now that you have identified your fun activity, give yourself permission to keep it in the schedule and enjoy it!

Action step

Write down three things you enjoyed doing as a child. Now identify three things that would really feel fun to you as an adult. Which of these could you realistically pencil into your schedule on a regular basis—and which would give you the most feelings of anticipation and excitement?

1. _____

2. _____

3. _____

Day 18

INSPIRATION: Where Did the Kid in You Go?

As business partners, we (Dr. Lerner and Dr. Loman) put on life-development camps called Camp Transformation. One of the purposes of the camp is to help participants explore their lives. We address many aspects, including desires, purpose, schedules, weaknesses, and other areas of life. At a recent camp, one of the doctors who attended was a little on the serious side. In fact, "a little" is being very nice. He was actually so serious that you very seldom saw a smile. He dressed ultra conservatively, and it seemed his facial expression was carved in stone.

His wife said, "He never has fun." She compared her husband's behavior after work every day to a robot. "He walks in the house, kisses me, says hi to the kids and goes into his office. Don't get me wrong; he is considered to be a great husband. In fact, he could get a 'Leader of the House' award."

At one point, I asked the doctor, "Do you ever come home and wrestle with your children or have a pillow fight?" He looked at me like I was speaking a foreign language. I instructed him to go home, wet down the lawn in the backyard and roll around in the mud. I also told him to bleach his hair blonde. "Just have some fun, Doc," I suggested. When I saw him at the next seminar, his face had changed. He actually had a smile on it! He was wearing a Hawaiian shirt and really had dyed his hair blonde. Oh, yeah! He did go wrestle with the kids in the yard. He was a new man. Actually, I take that back.

He was always that man, but for some reason life got hold of him and turned him into a very stoic, serious, and let's face it—boring—person.

The Bottom Line for Day 18

Lighten up! Make sure that the fun activity you chose in days 16 and 17 is really, truly fun, and I mean kid-like, goofy fun!

Action Step

Do your fun activity, and make it your goal to get as much out of it as you can. Laugh out loud!

> When a man has lost all happiness, he's not alive. Call him a breathing corpse.
> ~ Sophocles, ancient Greek playwright

Day 19

EXERCISE: These Shoes Were Made for Walking

Earlier in the Maximized Living Makeover challenge we began to explore exercise as something that can be fun. We also began to show you that exercise can be as simple as walking more by parking farther away from your destination. How have you been doing?

If you haven't been implementing your earlier action steps or you are starting to slide, get back on track. Review the first eighteen days, and let's keep rolling down the track toward maximized living. So if you have not been parking in the farthest spot from the front door of your destination, do it today.

The next step in moving this body is to take a few more "first steps." The steps I am talking about here are not only the literal steps; they are also the steps you need to take to make new behavior into a habit. For many things in life, to gain a new perspective you need to step into someone else's shoes. To make new exercise habits, you need to step into your own shoes. Today, take the time to go buy yourself a new pair of shoes. Not dress shoes. (That could have been your fun activity yesterday, but that's not what we mean today!) Today, go purchase a pair of good walking or running shoes.

Please do not think, "I can't afford them." You *must* afford them. By walking, jogging, and getting your body moving more, you will prevent heart disease and save yourself hundreds of thousands of dollars. (Remember our inspiration from day 2?) That means in the long run, these shoes will actually pay you. You also deserve that great feeling you get when you walk out of a store with something new. If you are a shopaholic, tell your twelve-step instructor it is for your health.

Isn't that going to be a great feeling to walk out of the store with new shoes that are going to change your life? Make sure that after you purchase them, you go straight home and take a long walk. At this point of the Maximized Living Makeover, you should start to focus on scheduling some exercise—oops, sorry, *moving* the body more. Get the right shoes, put them on, and use them to get yourself moving!

The Bottom Line for Day 19

New walking or running shoes are necessary to get you in gear to move your body more.

Action Step

Buy new shoes and take a walk.

> Progress is the sum of small victories won by individual human beings.
> ~ *Bruce Catton, Pulitzer Prize–winning journalist and historian*

Day 20

EXERCISE: Find Some Company

> Victory is won not in miles, but in inches. Win a little now, hold your ground, and later win a little more.
> ~ *Louis L'Amour, award-winning author*

So how are you doing today? We have made it through nineteen days. I hope you are proud of yourself. I hope all is going well for you. If you haven't followed the action steps perfectly, that's just fine. Pat yourself on the back for the days that you have. Then keep going. Let yesterday be yesterday and tomorrow be tomorrow. It does not matter what did or did not happen yesterday, and it does not matter what will or will not happen tomorrow. Concentrate on day 20 today.

Today you are starting a fresh, new life. And this fresh, new life includes moving more. At times, moving the body by yourself is lonely. The ability to self-motivate can often be one the most difficult acts as a human being. Right at this moment there are probably hundreds of thousands of people procrastinating about exercising. (OK, we're going to use the "e" word—*exercise*—sometimes. You can take it.) I am willing to bet that I am grossly underestimating the true number. Even top athletes procrastinate sometimes.

We all need a little help. If you have not already found a partner to move with, today is the day. It is OK, healthy even, to recognize that you need help making it through the Challenge. I am not going to ask you to go hire a trainer. All I am going to ask is that today you call someone to partner with you. Ask them to take a walk with you or meet you at the park for a short bicycle ride today. Let them know you are struggling and you need some company.

Here are some suggestions for moving your body with a friend in tow:

1. Go for a walk with your dog.
2. Walk or ride a bike with your family or a friend.
3. Get your children away from TV or video games and walk to the corner or around the block.
4. Meet a friend at the beach or lake. Walking in sand is great for your legs!
5. Meet a friend at the mall and walk around the inside of it two times before you allow yourself to enter a store.

The Bottom Line for Day 20

Exercise loves company. It's a lot easier to keep yourself moving if you do it with a friend, family member, coworker, or even the dog!

Action Step

Find a friend to exercise with and start moving—today.

Day 21

EXERCISE: I Don't Have Time

> Time is like a river of fleeting events, and its current is strong: as soon as something comes into sight, it is swept past us, and something else takes its place and that too will be swept away.
>
> ~ Marcus Aurelius, ancient Roman emperor and philosopher

One of the biggest mistakes we can allow to happen is losing our mind (and our determination to keep going) if we miss a "moving the body" time. The second biggest mistake is to get depressed over such a simple issue. Finally, the largest mistake is to be unable to adapt to the moment.

Let me show you what I mean. If you have decided to get up early and meet a friend for a walk and the alarm does not go off, don't panic. And don't give up. It's going to be OK. There is nothing wrong with changing the time and walking at a different time. Your friend will probably understand. It is also completely acceptable (and actually preferable) to keep the appointment—just shorten it—if you haven't slept through all the time you had. The important thing to remember is that at the moment of crisis do not tell yourself that you do not have time. Your walking time can be reduced from thirty minutes down to ten or fifteen. It can also be moved to after work, in the evening, on your lunch hour, or during a break.

In fact, walking at lunchtime is a great time to get exercise into your schedule, and it is often a time when others would be happy to join you. In a few days, our nutrition section will talk about packing a lunch to ensure healthy eating. You can get your walk in for the day by bringing your clothes and walking shoes to work and taking fifteen minutes of your lunch hour to walk.

At this point of the Maximized Living Makeover, remind yourself that you have come too far to let one bad moment (or even several) get to you. Be OK with a little change in the schedule. Just stay focused on your overall challenge, and you will begin to make moving a habit. Before you know it, your life will be even further down the path to becoming healthier and happier—and that's maximized living!

Here are some ideas to help you fit walking time into your schedule:

1. If you work, take shoes with you so you can walk during your lunch break.
2. If you go to college, walk during the break between classes.
3. If have too much scheduled to fit walking in at all, drop something and put walking in its place. You can do it!

The Bottom Line for Day 21

Make moving-your-body time a must-do in your schedule, and don't give it up when glitches come.

Action Step

Find time to walk. Adjust your schedule if you hit a bump in the road, but don't give up!

Day 22

STRESS MANAGEMENT: You Management

> Not being able to govern events, I govern myself.
> ~ *Michel de Montaigne I, French Renaissance writer*

All too often, we let our environment get the best of us. What do I mean by our environment? I mean anything that is outside of our control. If you think about it, most of our daily stresses are out of our control. The reason today's plan of action is entitled "You Management" is simple: You must stop looking outside of yourself and seeing the situation as the cause of your stress. It is not the outside stress that is the problem; it is how you respond to it.

The reason this topic excites me so much is that little word *control*. I love control. You cannot control the weather; however, you sure can control how you respond to the weather (you management). You can't control whether or not your two-year-old will throw a temper tantrum in the middle of the grocery store line. You can control how you react to it (you management). See what I mean?

Life becomes very stressful when you believe that you are merely like a sailboat without a rudder, drifting aimlessly wherever the wind blows you. When the wind changes, so do you. This way of thinking sets you up for stress. The idea of not having any control of the outcome of your life is stressful in and of itself.

Today's point is to take a look at the little frustrations in your life that bother you the most. Maybe it is crazy drivers who cut you off or traffic in general. Maybe it is your former spouse, your current boss, or the mind-numbing chores you have to do as a stay-at-home mom. As you look at what you do every day and pinpoint the areas that bother you the most, think about the way you react to them. Do you yell and scream at people, take your frustrations out by grounding your kids for the slightest infractions, or internalize all the irritation until you think you are going to explode?

Now that you have identified the things that really drive you to distraction and thought about your own reactions, remember this: you can't control the things that drive you crazy, but you *can* change your reactions to them. Determine to do things differently. If traffic makes you tense, stop and take a few deep breaths, say a prayer, or take a minute or two of quiet time just before you hit the road. If your boss drives you crazy, go out of your way to be the best employee you can be, and remember what you tell your kids, "Just because someone else is being mean, doesn't mean you can act that way to them."

If house chores are driving you nuts, get rid of the irritation by putting on your favorite music while you mop, assigning your least favorites to your older children, or trading a day of housecleaning with a friend (where you clean her house together one day a week, then switch to your house on a different day. It's amazing how much more fun it is to clean someone else's place!)

The Bottom Line for Day 22

You can rarely control your circumstances, but you can always control your reactions to the circumstances.

Action Step

Write down three things that cause you the most frustration and the ways you typically react. Now list one way you can change your reaction to each of these stressors, and try it.

1. _____

2. _____

3. _____

Day 23

STRESS MANAGEMENT: Schedule Management

On any given, overpacked day, the average American is about one task away from a straightjacket. I bet there are not too many days that you get to wake up and remain in bed resting for the first ten to thirty minutes. I am not talking about hitting the snooze alarm and going back to sleep. After all, you just slept for eight hours if you have allotted the Maximized Living amount of sleep to refresh yourself, right?

I am talking about taking the first few minutes of the day to get your mind prepared for what lies ahead. Take time to meditate and visualize your day. Note that I did not say stress over your day. This is time you allow your body to wake up and get mentally ready for the day.

I know you do not have time for that, but this is why we have this point as day 23 in the Maximized Living Makeover. Hear me out. I suspect that, every morning, your day has to begin. I am also betting that you may already feel like you are behind by a couple of hours from the moment you open your eyes. There is too much to do and too little time to get it done. As you are first waking up, your brain is already racing, worrying about the day. Maybe the reason you are so cranky and irritated at the traffic is that every morning you feel like you've already been behind since 6:00 a.m.

Instead of allowing your tasks ahead to dictate your emotions, take the time when you first wake up each morning to delete yesterday and not think about tomorrow—just get ready for today. Relax for your first fifteen minutes and get your mind, heart, and body ready for a great day.

The Bottom Line for Day 23

Staying in bed for a few extra minutes each morning to get mentally and emotionally prepared for the day can prevent stress and frustration during the day.

Action Step

Wake up fifteen minutes early and spend some time by yourself. Sit back and look at the sunrise or the stars and smile. Take this quiet time to relax and prepare for the day without feeling like you are already behind.

Day 24

STRESS MANAGEMENT:
Schedule Management: Lighten Your Load

The day is still only twenty-four hours long. As much as you would like there to be a way to lengthen each day, there are still only twenty-four hours. As we mentioned before, technology is doing everything it can to help us get more accomplished in each of our twenty-four hours. For example, with today's "toys":

1. We can do business on cell phones while driving down the road.
2. We can work on our laptops while we are flying on commercial flights.
3. We can send e-mails through our phones and computers.
4. We can hold business meetings through computer podcasting.
5. We can put our car on cruise control with radar so you do not run into the vehicle in front of you. (This way, you can turn around and reprimand your children while driving. Now that's multitasking!)

The list goes on and on. We can get a tremendous amount accomplished in a workday. However, this disease of accomplishing more is creating stress. I would almost call it a new disease. Maybe it should be called accomplish-itis or never-enough-itis.

The bottom line is our days are too full. Ten years ago, the average American slept eight hours each night. Now, we sleep less than seven hours. We are obviously trying to get more accomplished in life. But this is definitely one area where more does not mean better. More stress is never better, even if you are technically "getting more done." Eventually, the stress will cause such mental or physical breakdowns that it will cost you far more time, money and productivity than it would if you just slow down.

It is time to start looking at your schedule and identifying what needs to be taken out, chopped off at the knees or delegated to someone else. Here are the areas you should examine:

1. Your social life
2. Your work load
3. The chores you do
4. Your areas of volunteer service
5. Your obligations to family and friends

After you have examined each area, make a list of everything you do in each area. Prioritize them in order of how much time they take, the benefits you receive from doing them, and how much you enjoy them. Determine to eliminate the items that are at the bottom of each of your categories. Don't be afraid to say no to tasks that don't meet your criteria of benefit to you or your relationships. Get your schedule in order, and your burden of stress will be a lot lighter.

The Bottom Line for Day 24

Lightening your overloaded schedule will add much-needed peace to your life.

Action Step

Get something out of your schedule today that is causing too much stress. List three of the "bottom of the category" obligations you wrote down above. Choose the one that can go, and take it out of your schedule today!

1. _____

2. _____

3. _____

Day 25

NUTRITION: Relax, You Can Still Go to Wendy's

At this point in the Maximized Living Makeover, you should be well on your way to forming new, healthy habits and eliminating some of the old, unhealthy ones. You are on the path to great changes that lead to Maximized Living. You have received action points in the areas of inspiration, exercise, time management, nutrition, and stress management. Of these five, other than exercise I believe that nutrition and eating habits are the hardest to change. Change they must, but as we have pointed out before, we are not going to take your old eating habits and ask you to change every one of them in thirty days. So here's our top priority for today:

You can still go to your favorite fast-food restaurant!

You can go there, but what you order should start to change a little bit. At this point of the training, you know enough to begin to make smarter decisions about the fuel that you are putting into your body. Due to our fast-paced lives and crazy work schedules, it is inevitable that we begin to cut corners, especially in the area of food, as we hit the fast-food chains. But today's lesson is simple: if you must continue to eat at fast-food restaurants, take one or two of the items on the menu you would normally order and replace them with healthier items.

The first item I would evaluate is your choice of beverage. I know this one may hurt a little, but you can do it. Just try it. Do not order a soda. Instead, order bottled water. The amount of calories we are putting in to our bodies through high fructose, corn syrup–filled or sugar-laden liquids is astounding.

Remember that 75 to 85 percent of your body is water. One of the reasons you have decreased energy is due to dehydration. Most Americans are dehydrated.

Sodas compound the problem. The chemicals in soda actually remove water from your body, so you need to drink extra water for each soda you ingest. Therefore, ordering water the next time you hit McDonald's or Wendy's is a relatively painless way to make a great change in your health.

The Bottom Line for Day 25

You can still go to the restaurants you love, but get creative in replacing at least one unhealthy item with a healthier choice.

Action Step

Replace an unhealthy item with a healthier item. Here are some examples:
1. Replace a soda with water.
2. Replace French fries with a salad.
3. Eat two hamburgers and leave out the French fries.
4. Replace French fries with chili.
5. Order only salad, water, and maybe a dessert.

Day 26

NUTRITION: Protect Your Environment

I do not believe I have met anyone who is not influenced by his environment. The people who begin to master their lives are the ones who begin to overcome their environment more than they did the year before. Nutritionally, your environment can be identified by many situations. Imagine that you are at work, and it is time to take your lunch. There is not much time and a friend says, "We only have thirty minutes. Where do you want to go?" If there is food within walking distance, it is typically fast food. At this moment the environment is going to win. Now think of break time at work or snack time with the kids. When you see a vending machine or ice cream shop and you are hungry, who's going to win—your will or the environment?

Your environment in this situation is time, distance, and ease, along with fast food on every corner. As much as you want to eat a little healthier, your environment is probably going to win. The question is: Are you going to put up with that?

Wouldn't you like to win in these situations? Me, too. The great thing is you *can* win. It just takes a little preparation. Don't worry; I am not going to ask you to starve. The way you win when faced with these temptations is to think ahead. Bring your own lunches and snacks. I know what you are thinking. Immediately, you get a flashback of your elementary years when mom always packed you the worst food on the planet. I would choose starvation most of the time. I also know that you could not wait until you were big and you could buy your own food. This pattern from childhood has scarred you for life.

To resolve this painful psychosis, boycott the fast-food restaurant and vending machine at least once a week and pack your favorite lunch—one that you have chosen. Also, take time to buy some healthy, tasty snacks that you love. Bring them with you when you are at work or on the road. You'll be glad you did!

> What saves a man is to take a step. Then take another.
> ~ Antoine de Saint Exupéry, author, *The Little Prince*

The Bottom Line for Day 26

You can choose to protect your nutritional environment by being prepared for temptations along the way. Pack your lunch and snacks!

Action Step

Develop the lunch of your dreams. Remember, it must be healthy. Go to a grocery store like Wild Oats or Whole Foods and find some fun foods that you will enjoy. Ask for help and buy some healthy snacks too.

Day 27

TIME MANAGEMENT: 168-Hour Week

Have you ever added up the week and identified how many hours you have to work with? Don't worry; most people haven't. Just so you know, there are 168 hours in a week—and how we use those hours will determine our happiness. Our use of the time given to us governs our success. We must know what can be accomplished in a week in a healthy manner if we don't want to commit ourselves to a rehabilitation center.

The greatest way to identify if you are wasting time or have just lost time in your week is to literally lay out each hour. After doing this drill for years, there are two very distinctive outcomes. Both are on opposite sides of the spectrum of time usage.

After the drill, you will clearly see that you have too much scheduled and it is time to cut the fat.

OR

After the drill, you will look at your week and think, "Where am I wasting all that time?" You may have ten to twenty-five hours of time that is not accounted for.

Try it now. Lay out your schedule for a typical week—even this week—and see where your time is spent.

The Bottom Line for Day 27

You can recover time in your week by examining each hour to see where you are wasting time or pinpoint places where you are overcommitted.

Action Step

Break down your week and see where your time is spent.

168-HOUR WEEK		
_____ Sleep	_____ Eating	_____ Hygiene
_____ Work	_____ Chores	_____ Family Time
_____ Exercise	_____ Church/Bible Time	_____ TV
_____ Recreation	_____ Private Time	

Add up the hours you engage in each category daily. Then multiply by seven. If there is not a category above for some of your activities, develop an additional category or put that activity in an existing category. Add up all the hours and identify how much time you waste or how overscheduled your life has become.

Day 28

EXERCISE: Change Your Mind

At this point of the Maximized Living Makeover challenge, it is time to stop seeing yourself as a beginner. You have purchased your shoes and hopefully some fancy new walking clothes, and you are walking farther than you have before. I suspect it is going well.

> To do anything in this world worth doing, we must not stand back shivering and thinking of the cold and danger, and jump in and scramble through as well as we can.
>
> ~ Sydney Smith, English essayist

Now it is time to begin to move to the next level of exercise. You no longer see it as a bad word. The fear of acting has completely left your consciousness. So how much more energy do you have? I'm sure you are sleeping better, right? With the positive changes we've made throughout this challenge, you feel better about yourself. I'll bet you are beginning to see life in a different light.

It is time to start moving your body more. It is time to move from walking to starting to add time intervals where you will jog for short periods. For many, the idea of jogging is painful. I understand. Embarrassment sets in; uncertainty and fear that you may hurt yourself begin to overwhelm you. Some may have age issues, functional issues when frankly, they never have jogged in their life.

This moment is historic for you. But we are faced with moments in life where we can walk through a door and become something different, or we can re-live our same weakness and issues. It is time to no longer see yourself as a person who does not like to work out. It is time to no longer see yourself as too old. It is time to allow yourself to become a more powerful person and break out of the old level of thinking that has caused you to be held back in life.

Do not allow your past experiences to dictate who you are today or what you are willing to do today.

The Bottom Line for Day 28

You are more powerful than you think, and you are capable of moving more. Change your mind-set, and change your life!

Action Step

Call your walking partner and let them know that the team will add small periods of jogging. Walk for five minutes and jog for thirty seconds. Repeat this for thirty minutes. I know you can do it!

Day 29

INSPIRATION: Why Do You Wake Up?

Wow, only one more day! At this point, you should have made definite, visible changes in your life. You are feeling good, and you are beginning to see life through a different perspective.

Have you ever noticed that some people diet, exercise and enter into programs, then ultimately end up where they started? Maybe you have been on that roller coaster ride. But this challenge is different. It is one you can continue for life, because it is all about adding positive changes, not taking away the things you think you love.

As we close up the beginner section to the Maximized Living Makeover there is still one vital topic to discuss. Those who experience a truly fulfilled life have a purpose. They wake up every day with a reason to live. These people have decided to make a positive contribution to humanity.

Having a purpose is more than a job, more than raising a family, more than some day buying that fishing boat and retiring. A purpose is something that is bigger than you. In fact, your life's purpose cannot be about you. It must be about serving something bigger and outside of you.

Purpose fulfills that missing piece that you sometimes feel is empty. That empty part of your soul cannot be filled with diamonds, cars, boats, vacations, vacation homes or even the man or woman of your dreams. None of those will fit into that vault. The only way to fill that missing part of you is to find the reason you wake up each morning.

Identify your passion and you will be a lot closer to figuring out your purpose. What activities do you enjoy doing for others the most? What injustices hurt you the most or make you feel the most upset? What wrongs in the world would you like to see righted? There are many ways that you can reach out to those around you and leave a positive legacy long after you are gone. Start reaching out today, and identify your life's purpose.

The Bottom Line for Day 29

Take time to identify your true purpose in life, the way you can reach out and make a positive difference in this world. You won't feel truly fulfilled until you do!

Action Step

Take time to identify your purpose. The larger the purpose, the larger life will be for you.

Day 30

INSPIRATION: The Rest of Your Life

Congratulations! You made it! Have you thought about what you have done? At this point, you have completed the thirty-day Maximized Living Beginners Makeover Challenge. But we hesitate in making that statement.

At this point you should not see this as a point where you are finished. Life is never finished. The last twenty-nine days should be looked at as a twenty-nine-day program to prepare you for the positive changes you will keep making for the rest of your life.

Imagine looking forward ten, twenty or even fifty years from now and still living the Maximized Living lifestyle. This is a reality that is up to you. People who work out, eat healthy, and strive for a better life did not wake up after twenty years and discover that they accidentally ended up there. These people decided to do something different and acted upon that decision.

For the last twenty-nine days you have been preparing for this moment. This is the moment—today—that you get to decide to continue the lifestyle you have started. It's a lifestyle that will give you abundant life and millions of dollars. (Remember, living this lifestyle saves you money and misery in the long run!)

The Bottom Line for Day 30

Congratulations! You made it! Now keep it going for life!

Action Step

Keep making healthy and positive choices each day, and keep watching yourself transform into the fulfilled, healthy person you were created to be.

INTERMEDIATE AND ELITE
MAKEOVER CHALLENGES

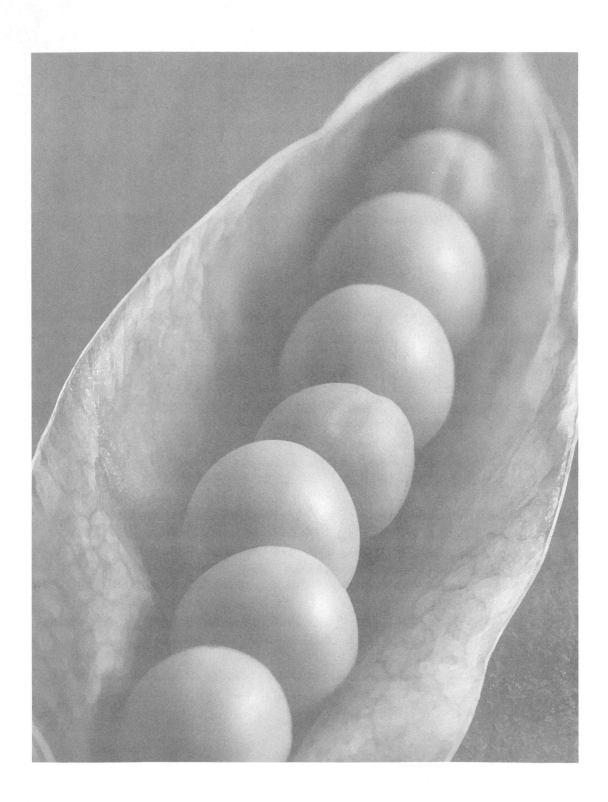

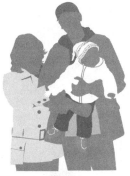

Day 1

Figure Out Where You Are

Self-examination is a necessity of life. The Maximized Living Intermediate Makeover Challenge begins by challenging you to take inventory of where you stand right now, today, on your path to maximized living. Do a self-assessment as to where you are, physically (weight, fitness levels, and overall health), mentally (attitude, temper, peace of mind, emotions), relationships (marriage, kids, other family members, friends, coworkers), financially (debt, financial peace, direction, overall wealth), purpose (do you feel you spend your life focused on making the difference you were born to make?), passion (are you excited about your life?). Finally, ask yourself if you are having fun and doing what you love to do. You can use the space below or start a journal or notebook to go along with your intermediate journey.

_____

_____

_____

_____

Now take a few minutes to think about your dreams. What are your goals? Where do you see yourself in the future? (i.e. goals for the areas being examined above—physical, mental, relational, financial, purpose, direction, and fun). Record your thoughts here or in your journal.

_____

_____

_____

_____

If you were living life to the max, what would that look like?

_____

_____

_____

_____

_____

_____

_____

Measure on a scale of 1 to 10 (1 = Terrible, 10 = Excellent)

Overall health

| 1 | 2 | 3 | 4 | 5 | 6 | 7 | 8 | 9 | 10 |

Energy level

| 1 | 2 | 3 | 4 | 5 | 6 | 7 | 8 | 9 | 10 |

Stress level

| 1 | 2 | 3 | 4 | 5 | 6 | 7 | 8 | 9 | 10 |

Attitude (Are you generally happy and positive?)

| 1 | 2 | 3 | 4 | 5 | 6 | 7 | 8 | 9 | 10 |

Time management skills

| 1 | 2 | 3 | 4 | 5 | 6 | 7 | 8 | 9 | 10 |

Spouse/significant other relationship

| 1 | 2 | 3 | 4 | 5 | 6 | 7 | 8 | 9 | 10 |

Relationship with kids

| 1 | 2 | 3 | 4 | 5 | 6 | 7 | 8 | 9 | 10 |

Relationships with others

| 1 | 2 | 3 | 4 | 5 | 6 | 7 | 8 | 9 | 10 |

Financial stability

| 1 | 2 | 3 | 4 | 5 | 6 | 7 | 8 | 9 | 10 |

On course to finding and/or fulfilling your mission in life

| 1 | 2 | 3 | 4 | 5 | 6 | 7 | 8 | 9 | 10 |

Adult Body Mass Index

$$BMI = \left[\frac{WEIGHT\ (pounds)}{Height\ (inches)^2}\right] \times 703$$

HEIGHT IN FEET & INCHES \ WEIGHT IN POUNDS	120	130	140	150	160	170	180	190	200	210	220	230	240	250
4'-6"	29	31	34	36	39	41	43	46	48	51	53	56	58	60
4'-8"	27	29	31	34	36	38	40	43	45	47	49	52	54	56
4'-10"	25	27	29	31	34	36	38	40	42	44	46	48	50	52
5'-0"	23	25	27	29	31	33	35	37	39	41	43	45	47	49
5'-2"	22	24	26	27	29	31	33	35	37	38	40	42	44	46
5'-4"	21	22	24	26	28	29	31	33	34	36	38	40	41	43
5'-6"	19	21	23	24	26	27	29	31	32	34	36	37	39	40
5'-8"	18	20	21	23	24	26	27	29	30	32	34	35	37	38
5'-10"	17	19	20	22	23	24	26	27	29	30	32	33	35	36
6'-0"	16	18	19	20	22	23	24	26	27	28	30	31	33	34
6'-2"	15	17	18	19	21	22	23	24	26	27	28	30	31	32
6'-4"	15	16	17	18	20	21	22	23	24	26	27	28	29	30
6'-6"	14	15	16	17	19	20	21	22	23	24	25	27	28	29
6'-8"	13	14	15	17	18	19	20	21	22	23	24	25	26	28

■ Healthy Weight   ■ Overweight   ■ Obese

Now get out the dreaded scale and a tape measure and record your body weight and measurements as follows. You will also need to get your most recent blood work reports from your doctor or laboratory or have blood work done if you haven't had it done in more than a year.

		Cholesterol		Body measurements	
	Weight		Total		Chest
	Percentage of body fat		HDL		Upper arm
	Blood pressure		LDL		Upper thigh
			Other important blood counts		Waist

The next step in day 1 of the Intermediate Makeover Challenge is centered around Essential 4: maximize lean muscle and oxygen. Today you will begin the basic SURGE training program (described in chapter 6). This week, plan to follow the SURGE program for four days, for a total of twelve minutes of exercise. Here is how you do it:

Basic SURGE Program

The first step is to calculate your training zone.

Your maximum heart rate (MHR) = 220 – your age.

After your SURGE, your heart rate should be in the 75 to 85 percent range of your MHR. (Grab a calculator, and take your maximum heart rate number and multiply it times .75 and .85 to determine your range.)

- Increase by five beats if you are regularly exercising.
- Increase by ten beats if you are an experienced athlete.
- Lower by five beats if you are just starting.
- Lower by ten beats if you are on medication or recovering from injury or illness.

⚡Note: Elite athletes can train at or even above the MHR following a SURGE.

You can find your heartbeat simply by placing your fingers lightly but firmly over the inside of your wrist or on your neck, just below the angle of your jaw. (CAUTION: Do not put too much pressure on the neck; this can slow the heart down, make you dizzy, cause you to lose consciousness, and can be dangerous for anyone with potential blockages of blood vessels in the neck.)

Another way to monitor your heartbeat is to put your hand over your heart and count the number of beats or simply use a heart monitor, which is available at any sporting goods store.

WARNING: Consult your doctor before beginning this program. If your heart rate goes up too high following a SURGE, reduce the SURGE time. If it still goes too high or actually jumps up, consult your physician.

SURGE training can be done using a stepper, stepping up and down on a step, or simply stepping up and down in place on the floor as fast as you can. This can also be done while lifting a weight from your side, up and over your head to add resistance into the movement. Here is an example of one SURGE cycle:

One SURGE Cycle

- Twenty seconds on (Heart rate up to the training zone)
- Twenty seconds off (Full recovery time to get heart rate back to the bottom of the training zone or below)
- Twenty seconds on
- Twenty seconds off
- Twenty seconds on
- Twenty seconds off (Don't cheat on time here; recovery is important for full SURGE effect.)
- Repeat this cycle three to four times for three to four minutes of total exercise or approximately twelve to fifteen minutes total elapsed time.

Total exercise time for an entire week on the basic SURGE program is only twelve to sixteen minutes, and total elapsed time for an entire week is an hour or less! Remember, with the SURGE program, no one can use time as an excuse now for not getting healthy and in the best shape of your life!

More advanced athletes can work this into their weekly training and/or increase the number of SURGES per session to radically improve their performance times. They can also add on to the twenty seconds up to sixty-second surges max, but never going beyond a peak output.

Now that you have assessed where you stand, considered your overall health, and completed your first SURGE, it's time to focus on Essential 5: maximize peace and strong relationships. Maximize peace by writing out your To-do list for this first week so that you are not memory managing but instead have everything written down that needs to be accomplished this week, as well as what day and time you will accomplish it.

Action Steps

1. Fill out your self-assessment.
2. Do your SURGE.
3. Write out your To-do list along with specific times and days of accomplishment.

To Add the Elite Makeover Challenge

If you are already a seasoned athlete, a professional athlete, a health foods "nut" in really good shape, or if you have completed the Maximized Living Intermediate Makeover Challenge (maybe even more than once), you are ready to move into the ranks of the elite. Also, if you're sick and really want to get well and/or really committed to your health—the Elite Makeover Challenge is for you. Welcome to the Maximized Living Elite Makeover Challenge.

For the next thirty days, you will continue to follow all of the steps, rules, and plans outlined in the Intermediate Makeover Challenge, but each day of the Elite Makeover Challenge will take you just a little bit farther down the path toward the full realization of Maximized Living. If you are a seasoned or professional athlete and jumped right to this Elite Makeover Challenge, be sure you continue to follow the Intermediate Makeover Challenge steps, rules, and game plans that have already been established in all areas of the Five Essentials.

Congratulations on the hard work you have already done to get your mind, body, and emotions in top working order! Now, get ready to go to the next level with the Elite Makeover Challenge!

Elite Makeover Challenge

Day 1

Assess Yourself

Before you begin the day-by-day steps, it's very important that you assess where you are right now. Only by taking stock of where you stand at the beginning can you look back at the end and see how far you've come. So today's action step is the same as it is for the Intermediate Makeover Challenge: Assess yourself.

Action Steps

Fill out your self-assessment in the Intermediate Makeover Challenge.
- ESSENTIAL 4 ACTION: Do your SURGE.
- ESSENTIAL 5 ACTION: Write out a To-do list along with specific times and days of accomplishment.

Intermediate Makeover Challenge

Day 2

Food Makes an Impact on Your Future

The American people are now more overweight than ever, childhood obesity has tripled, and nutritionally related diseases are at an all-time high. As the Western diet is adopted overseas, these problems follow close behind. The issue isn't an epidemic of big pants and long belts – it's an epidemic of disease in overwhelming proportions. Additionally, the modern diet is nutrient-deficient. Therefore, we're overweight but actually undernourished.

Why is this important to note? Because having a high BMI or being even moderately overweight and/or or having a diet deficient in important key elements is linked to almost every disease and cause of death. The foods you eat make a huge impact on your future. Max foods, as discussed in chapter 5, are the foods that create the best opportunity for maximized living and maximized health.

Max-Foods List

Max foods include fruits, whole grains, vegetables, proteins (eggs, fish and chicken), good fats (like avocado, almonds, and olive oil), and all kinds of nuts and seeds. These live foods can all be made into hundreds, if not thousands, of easy recipes that will make you never miss anything or have cravings. (And if you do miss something, remember that you can schedule a "vacation meal.")

As we stated in the Beginner Makeover Challenge, cutting foods out of your daily diet is not the way to start a healthier lifestyle. Instead, start by using the addition rule and adding good things. For example, start eating an apple with your donut and coffee in the morning and a salad with your milkshake and fries at lunch.

See the complete Max foods list in chapter 5 for the best choices of foods to eat.

Action Steps

- ESSENTIAL 3 ACTION: Follow the addition rule today. Add a minimum of five foods from the Max foods list to your diet each day. Add one at breakfast, two at lunch (or one for a mid-morning snack and one at lunch), and two at dinner (or one as a mid-afternoon snack and one at dinner).
- ESSENTIAL 3 ACTION: Max Beginner Diet. Begin applying the three changes:
  1. Look for healthier meats.
  2. Start using only good fats.
  3. Become aware of your sugars and refined grains and begin to eliminate.

- ESSENTIAL 4 ACTION: SURGE
- ESSENTIAL 5 ACTION: Follow the To-do plan, cross off your accomplishments, and evaluate your schedule for tomorrow. Make adjustments as necessary.

Elite Makeover Challenge

Day 2
Fail to Plan = Plan to Fail

Goal setting can make the critical difference between success and failure. If you want abundance in every area of your life, you first have to be clear about what you want. Let me make that perfectly clear: You have to know exactly what you want. Goal setting is a powerful tool, whether it is applied to one's professional life, personal aspirations, or health objectives.

Your life may seem out of control at times, but you need to keep reminding yourself that you hold the greatest power of all. You have the ability to design your own life and the capability of enjoying the Maximized Living life you've always dreamed about. You can wake up every morning, meditate, exercise, eat a nutritious breakfast, and take all your supplements. Or you can make choices that may be detrimental to your emotional and physical health. Ultimately, the decision is yours and yours alone.

Action Steps

Continue to follow the action steps from the Intermediate Makeover Challenge.

- ESSENTIAL 3 ACTION: The Intermediate Max Diet
  1. Remember: Meet Fat Sally:
     Good meats
     Good fats
     Eliminate refined sugars and grains
  2. Make your midday meal your last meal of the day containing carbohydrates. Stop eating breads, rices, grains, sugars, and potatoes in the afternoon and evening. Make vegetables, proteins, fats, nuts, and seeds your afternoon and evening foods.
- ESSENTIAL 5 ACTION: Set long-term and short-term goals for each of your many "lives." (See Intermediate Makeover Challenge, Day 9.) These include your physical life, mental life, business life, relationships life, family life, and so on.

- ESSENTIAL 2 ACTION: Make sure you find a Maximized Living Doctor to have the most important test of your life done...a computerized nervous system scan and x-rays to see if you have subluxation.

Intermediate Makeover Challenge

Day 3
Begin the Three-Day Diet Diary

Because food makes such an impact on the quality and quantity of your life, it is essential to know what you are already eating. Believe it or not, most people do not realize what they are putting in their mouths each day. Only by recording everything you eat over a period of time can you truly evaluate the kinds of foods you are eating, the amount of food you are eating, and the moods you are experiencing before and after eating. In order for you to get a good picture of exactly where you stand, today we will begin a three-day diet diary.

Three-Day Diet Diary
Day 1
1. Record the time of all food, beverage, vitamin, or medication intake.
2. Record the approximate size and amount of each item.
3. Record why you are eating—bored, tired, hungry, social, business, time, depressed, etc.
4. Record how you felt after eating. How did you feel one hour after eating?
5. Please note if there is a time of day where you are particularly stressed, tired, or in a lot of pain.

_____

_____

_____

_____

Day 2
1. Record the time of all food, beverage, vitamin, or medication intake.
2. Record the approximate size and amount of each item.
3. Record why you are eating—bored, tired, hungry, social, business, time, depressed, etc.

4. Record how you felt after eating. How did you feel one hour after eating?
5. Please note if there is a time of day where you are particularly stressed, tired, or in a lot of pain.

_____

_____

_____

Day 3

1. Record the time of all food, beverage, vitamin, or medication intake.
2. Record the approximate size and amount of each item.
3. Record why you are eating—bored, tired, hungry, social, business, time, depressed, etc.
4. Record how you felt after eating. How did you feel one hour after eating?
5. Please note if there is a time of day where you are particularly stressed, tired, or in a lot of pain.

_____

_____

_____

Now write down your favorite Max foods that you could see putting in your diet every week. List them by category: fats, carbohydrates, or proteins.

_____

_____

_____

_____

_____

Action Steps

- ESSENTIAL 3 ACTION: Fill out day 1 of the three-day diet diary.
- ESSENTIAL 3 ACTION: Continue following the addition rule.
- ESSENTIAL 3 ACTION: Beginner Max Diet—"Meet Fat Sally"
- ESSENTIAL 5 ACTION: Follow your To-do plan, cross off accomplishments, and evaluate for tomorrow.

Elite Makeover Challenge

Day 3
Adopt an Attitude of Gratitude

Nothing new can come into your life until you're grateful for what you have. Today, and for the rest of your life, it's time to focus on all the great things in your life. We spend too much time thinking happiness will come after we achieve all our goals; however, the reality is that unless you're happy now, you will never be happy after you achieve more goals.

Action Steps

Continue all your action steps from the Intermediate Makeover Challenge.

- ESSENTIAL 3 ACTION: Intermediate Max Diet—"Meet Fat Sally" and no sugars, grains, or other carbs after midday.
- ESSENTIAL 5 ACTION: Make a list of everything you are grateful for in every aspect of your life. After you make that list, make sure it's part of what you read in your Peace Triathlon (See Intermediate Makeover Challenge, day 4) when you first wake up each morning.

Intermediate Makeover Challenge

Day 4
Build on What You've Started

On this fourth day of the Intermediate Makeover Challenge, it's time to keep building on what you've begun. You're off to a great start. Now it's time to keep hitting all the areas we've covered so far. It's the second day of your three-day diet diary, and you should keep adding Max foods to your diet today. Head to the store and pick up some you've never tried before, or pull out some old favorites. You'll SURGE again today, and we'll add a new action point for maximizing peace and strong relationships.

So what are you waiting for? Read today's action steps and get started!

Action Steps

- ESSENTIAL 3 ACTION: Fill out day 2 of your three-day diet diary.
- ESSENTIAL 3 ACTION: Continue following the Addition Rule and adding Max foods to your diet today.

⚡Note: Day 7 is the day you can apply the vacation rule. On this day, you can have any or all of your favorite food(s) with no guilt! This should help you stick to better, Max foods the rest of the week, because you know you can satisfy your cravings soon.

- ESSENTIAL 3 ACTION: Keep following the Beginner Max Diet.
- ESSENTIAL 4 ACTION: Do your SURGE.
- ESSENTIAL 5 ACTION: Start the daily Peace Triathlon right when you get up today, and try to make a habit of doing it every day.

⚡Note: The Peace Triathlon may require getting up fifteen minutes earlier than usual. If you're a snooze button hitter, set the alarm twenty-four minutes earlier.

Here are the components of the Peace Triathlon:
1. Observe five minutes of silence. Keep your mind empty; try to let no thoughts enter. (See also meditation in chapter 7)
2. Practice five minutes of visualization. Focus on how you want to positively and proactively respond to the day's events. Picture yourself acting out mental and emotional control, even in difficult situations.
3. Finish with five minutes of reading. Choose positive, inspiring, and empowering literature like a devotional, personal development book, biography of a strong and courageous person, or the Bible.

- ESSENTIAL 5 ACTION: Follow your To-do list, cross off your accomplishments, and evaluate for tomorrow.

Elite Makeover Challenge

Day 4
Check Your (pH) Balance

Your body's pH should be neutral (7.0). If it's under that, you are acidic. Viruses, bacteria, funguses, and almost all diseases grow in acidic environments. It's important to know whether you are balanced. Check your pH and determine if you need to make changes to keep your body chemistry balanced. In order to check your pH you need to order pH strips. Read more at www.MaximizedLivingMakeover.com

If you have severe need of healing from disease, toxicity, pain, inflammation, or high cholesterol/high blood pressure, then begin moving toward the Advanced Healing Diet (Max Elite).

You can look back in chapter 5 for a refresher on the Advanced Healing Diet. For the Elite Max Diet, remember: How Sally Got So Fat

1. **NO SUGARS** – Sally
2. **NO GRAINS** – Got
3. **FATS** – Fat
4. **NO FRUITS** – From
5. **PROTEIN** – Pumpernickel

Basically, the Elite Max Diet eliminates all sugars and anything that the body turns to sugar (grains), emphasizing fats, protein, and vegetables.

Action Steps

Continue all your action steps from the Intermediate Makeover Challenge.
- ESSENTIAL 3 ACTION: Follow the Intermediate or Advanced Healing Max Diet.
- ESSENTIAL 5 ACTION: Put on your attitude of gratitude.
- ESSENTIAL 1 ACTION: Start measuring your pH daily.
- ESSENTIAL 3 ACTION: Begin adding more alkaline foods and eliminating acidic foods from your diet. See alkaline/acidic foods at www.MaximizedLivingMakeover.com.

Intermediate Makeover Challenge

Day 5
Turn Resolutions into Revolutions

You do not stumble upon health and happiness; you *schedule* it. Time management turns resolutions into revolutions. Resolutions are typically broken by January 4. Revolutions can last a lifetime. But to have a revolution or real-life transformation, you have to plan. Time management creates consistency and real long-term change.

You hear an awful lot of people talk about "the good old days." This was a time long ago when people used to be in shape, follow an exercise program, read a lot, follow a "strict" diet, or be a great athlete. Apparently, at some point, "the good old days" became the "the bad new now" when knees and backs went bad, when babies were born, or when they got a job, got married, or got divorced.

Most nutrition plans, exercise programs, and stress management tools are like New Year's resolutions: their lifespan lasts only days. A few glorious days that many people will spend the rest of their lives saying, "I can remember when…"

At least six times out of ten, you will not feel like making healthy choices. Over half of the time, you will not be overly motivated to put in your nutrition time, exercise time, and even date times along with all of the other times necessary to attain maximized living.

The only reason you will follow and stick with the plan and do good things for your life and your body consistently for years to come is that, although you will not always feel like doing it, you will be *inspired* to do it

Pay close attention to this paragraph and re-read it, if necessary, to make sure that you really get it. *Motivation* is when it's about *you*. When you're motivated, you "feel like it." *Inspiration* is when it's about *others*. When your reason for doing something difficult is for the greater good of your family, your purpose, or mankind, you're more determined to follow through. When you're inspired, you're committed. And commitments are stronger than feelings. (We'll explore this further on day 24.)

Here's your inspiration mantra. Memorize it. Write it on a sticky note and post it on your mirror, or carry it with you in your wallet:

My commitment must be stronger than my feelings are at this moment.

Commit and the result will be that today—and all your days—will be "good old days."

Action Steps

- ESSENTIAL 3 ACTION: Follow the Big Four. No diet of any kind works without them. Here they are:

  1. SHOPPING: Write in time for shopping for Max foods. Making sure Max foods are available in the house is a big factor in your success. If all that's left is the stuff in the back of the cupboard or refrigerator—you're toast.
  2. COOKING: Cooking many meals at a time assures that you have good, quick foods always on hand. Prepared food, rather then food ripped open from a box or pried out of a can, is almost always the better food for you.
  3. PREPARING: If you will be gone during eating times, don't leave the house without some plastic containers filled with Max foods such as bags of nuts, raw vegetables, fruit, etc.
  4. PLANNING: Think ahead. Don't get stuck on an airplane, at work, or in your car hungry and without having Max foods available.

- ESSENTIAL 3 ACTION: Fill out day 3 of the three-day diet diary.
- ESSENTIAL 3 ACTION: Continue following the addition rule. Eat one Max. food at breakfast, two at midday, and two in the late afternoon and evening.
- ESSENTIAL 3 ACTION: Max Beginner Diet.
- ESSENTIAL 5 ACTION: Continue the Peace Triathlon.

Elite Makeover Challenge

Day 5
Meditate On It

In chapter 7, you learned the importance of meditation (building mental muscle) and how to do it. This is a critical step to decreasing stress daily. The key is to focus on the most important person in your life, you. All success comes from the inside out. Go back to chapter 7 and practice doing the two meditations that were explained there. Learn how to build "mental muscle" through meditation at www.MaximizedLivingMakeover.com.

Action Steps

Continue all your action steps from the Intermediate Makeover Challenge.

- ESSENTIAL 5 ACTION: Put on your attitude of gratitude.
- ESSENTIAL 1 AND 3 ACTION: Check your pH balance, and eat alkaline foods.
- ESSENTIAL 3 ACTION: Intermediate Max Diet or eliminate sugars as you continue the Elite Max Diet.
- ESSENTIAL 5 ACTION: Decide what time every morning you're going to meditate. Put it on your To-do list. You can begin with ten minutes a day and work up to thirty minutes.

Intermediate Makeover Challenge

Day 6
Evaluate Your Diet Diary
Begin the Intermediate Max Diet

You've spent the last three days tracking every morsel of food that went into your mouth—and how you felt about it before and after you ate it. Now it's time to figure out what it all means. Today you are going to evaluate your three-day diet diary and begin the Intermediate Max Diet.

The first thing to notice is the types of foods you eat. Are you a carbaholic? Is sugar your main weakness? Next, look at the times of day when you eat the most. Evaluate what you were feeling at mealtimes. Were you driven to eat each meal by your body's hunger pangs, or did you eat some foods because they looked good, smelled good, were easy to grab or made you feel better?

By looking at your diet diary, you can tell a lot about what you are really eating, not what you think you have been eating. Many people think they eat better than they actually do, and a large number of Americans underestimate the amount of food they put into their bodies each day. We barely notice how many potato chips we ate in front of the TV last night or how many cookies followed lunch at our desks. By putting it down on paper, you have the cold, hard proof of how you truly eat.

Once you have examined your diet diary, you have a good foundation from which to make some changes. Take a look at how much of your food intake after 2:00 to 3:00 in the afternoon each day was in the grain and sugar carbohydrates category. This includes grains, flours, sugars, potatoes, rice, pasta, corn, peas, cereals, and breads. If you can eliminate these carbohydrates late in the day and through the evening, your body will be better off.

Working toward eliminating carbs after midday that either are sugar or turn into sugar after is the Intermediate Max Diet. Also, the best source of nutrients is from food. However, our foods no longer have the same amount of nutrients they did when we were younger. Today, it is crucial to do the basics, which means supplementing with a high-quality, multi-mineral vitamin daily.

Action Steps

- ESSENTIAL 3 ACTION: Start Intermediate Max Diet. Make the decision to eat only proteins, vegetables, nuts, seeds, and fats after 2:00 to 3:00 p.m.
- ESSENTIAL 3 ACTION: Begin taking your multivitamin with minerals.
- ESSENTIAL 3 ACTION: Continue the addition rule. You should now be eating a minimum of five Max foods a day, using proteins and fats from the Max-foods list in the afternoons and evenings.
- ESSENTIAL 4 ACTION: Don't forget to SURGE.
- ESSENTIAL 5 ACTION: Continue the Peace Triathlon each morning.
- ESSENTIAL 5 ACTION: Keep evaluating your To-do list, and strengthen it by giving action steps specific times to be accomplished.

Elite Makeover Challenge

Day 6

Alternate Your Exercises

In the Maximized Living Intermediate Makeover Challenge, you learned about the importance of SURGE training and how to do it. For the Elite Makeover Challenge, it's time to start setting goals and increasing your weights for resistance training, plus increasing your time during cardiovascular training (your SURGEs). If you do not have a home gym or exercise equipment of some kind, it's time to get some or become a member of a local gym, if you feel comfortable there. This will ensure that you are doing the appropriate workouts with the appropriate equipment. Go to www.MaximizedLivingMakeover.com to see how to do these exercises.

Action Steps

Continue all your action steps from the Intermediate Makeover Challenge.

- ESSENTIAL 5 ACTION: Put on your attitude of gratitude.
- ESSENTIAL 1 AND 3 ACTION: Check your pH balance and eat alkaline foods.
- ESSENTIAL 3 ACTION: Continue to follow the Intermediate or Elite Advanced Healing Max Diet.
- ESSENTIAL 5 ACTION: Meditate during your Peace Triathlon.
- ESSENTIAL 4 ACTION: Begin SURGE training six days on, one day off. Alternate cardio SURGES one day and Pause Sets the next day. Pause Sets equal one specific exercise each for chest, biceps, triceps, and abdominal muscles (abs), or one specific exercise each for legs (squats or lunges), calves, shoulders, and back/lateral muscles (lats). Each exercise takes only three minutes, for a total of ten to twelve minutes of exercise. For the Elite Makeover Challenge, aim to do two to three exercises per body part rather than just one to two like the intermediate. Pick a specific time of day that you know you will be able to maintain for consistency. The morning is the best time to work out.

Intermediate Makeover Challenge

Day 7
Use the Stay-Full and Multiple-Feedings Rule

Yesterday, you evaluated your food diary and discovered the ways you really eat. Then, you made the all-important decision to try no longer to eat grain and sugar carbohydrates from three o'clock in the afternoon on each day. But that's not an easy decision to keep, so today's new action step is to learn the stay-full and multiple-feedings rules.

The principles are simple. The stay-full rule means that you should keep yourself full of vegetables, proteins, and fats. That's where the multiple-feedings rule kicks in. In order to stay full, you need to eat multiple meals of the Max foods we just mentioned, by adding more meals in the late morning, mid-afternoon, and evening. This will make your cravings for sugar and carbohydrates manageable or may eliminate them altogether.

As you start to employ these new rules, we want to say "Congratulations!" for reaching the end of your first week of the Maximized Living Intermediate Makeover Challenge. You should already be seeing a positive difference in many areas of your life, especially in your eating habits, exercise habits, and state of mind and emotions. You are making wonderful adjustments to your life that will pay off for the rest of your life. And now that you've made it for a week, you get a vacation. Not from everything new you've learned, but a vacation day in your eating plan. Today you can eat the foods you've been craving all week (just try to get those carbohydrates and sugars in before three o'clock).

Action Steps

- ESSENTIAL 3 ACTION: Vacation meal! Eat the food or foods you've been craving all week. This is not only fun and something to look forward to, but also it will help you through the tough days.
- ESSENTIAL 3 ACTION: Use the stay-full and multiple-feeding rules. Stay full on the vegetables, proteins, and fats by adding more meals in the late morning, mid-afternoon, and evening so you do not crave sugars/carbohydrates.
- ESSENTIAL 3 ACTION: Continue following the addition rule. Eat one Max food at breakfast, two at midday, and two in the late afternoon and evening.
- ESSENTIAL 3 ACTION: Keep taking your multivitamin with minerals.
- ESSENTIAL 5 ACTION: Continue the Peace Triathlon.

Elite Makeover Challenge

Day 7

The Weekly Update

At the end of each week in the Elite Makeover Challenge, it is important to assess where you stand and what changes you have made.

Assess where you stand today by measuring and answering the following:

_____ New weight

_____ Body fat percent

_____ pH

_____ Blood pressure

_____ BMI

_____ How many days a week did you work out?

_____ How many days did you wake up with gratitude?

_____ How many days did you meditate?

Action Steps

Continue all your action steps from the Intermediate Makeover Challenge.
Assess where you stand today by looking back at where you were seven days ago.

- ESSENTIAL 1 AND 3 ACTION: Check your pH balance, and eat alkaline foods.
- ESSENTIAL 2 ACTION: Make sure you're staying on track with your chiropractic adjustments and at-home spinal corrective exercises.
- ESSENTIAL 3 ACTION: Follow the Intermediate and Advanced Healing Max Diets.
- ESSENTIAL 5 ACTION: Put on your attitude of gratitude.
- ESSENTIAL 5 ACTION: Meditate during your Peace Triathlon.

Intermediate Makeover Challenge

Day 8
Create a War Plan and Prioritize Your "Lives"

As you begin your second week of the Maximized Living Intermediate Makeover Challenge, it's time to get more specific with your To-do list. We call this your War Plan, and it will contain specific times allotted for each of your "lives." What do we mean by this?

Well, like cats, most of us have nine lives. Some of us have even more! Here's what we're talking about: You have a mental life where your thoughts take place, a family life, a fitness life, a life with your spouse, a parent life, a financial life, a purpose or mission life, a fun life, and a serious hobby life. What other lives do you have?

Each of these "lives" or categories of life need their own time and attention in order to remain viable. Yet many people live each life with no pre-planning to make sure the right lives get the right amount of attention. Today's new action step is to examine each of your lives and make a game plan—actually, a war plan—for serving them well.

Here are examples of the top five "lives" we live:
The Big 5 Lives
1. Spiritual life (praying, quiet time)
2. Family life (spouse, parent, relationships with friends and extended family)
3. Personal health and fitness life (movement and Food by Nature)
4. Your mission life (your purpose and passion)
5. Business or financial life (work, financial planning)

Once you have identified your own lives (you will list them below when you get to the action steps for today) and decided what needs to be accomplished in each, you need to write all of your action steps into your schedule. Set specific times for each item you need to add to your day and/or week. Write them in black ink so that you cannot erase them!

Examples
SHOPPING: Sunday at 3:00 p.m. or sometime in the afternoon
PREPARATION: Cook chicken and jasmine rice that can be taken to work for lunch for two or three days.
PREPARATION: Cook turkey breast from the grocery store on Monday night to use for kids' lunches on Tuesday and Wednesday.
EXERCISE: Monday/Wednesday/Thursday/Friday at noon do a lunchtime SURGE.

FAMILY:
- Monday at 5:30 p.m., craft time with five-year-old daughter
- Thursday at 7:00 p.m., babysitter arrives so you can have date time with spouse
- Friday at 6: p.m., bike ride with the family after dinner for twenty minutes
- Saturday at 9:00 a.m., shoot hoops with son at park or recreation center

By setting up your war plan, you are prepared to go into the battle for your time each day. You already know ahead of time what needs to be accomplished and when you are going to do it. This relieves a ton of stress and lets you rest easy knowing that you went beyond the "immediate" tasks, which can eat up your days, and went straight for the "important" items planned in your To-do list. Only with a war plan will you give yourself the time to stick to this makeover challenge and get closer to your goal of Maximized Living.

Answer the following questions:
Do you understand the battle you're engaged in? How can creating and following a war plan help you win?

_____

_____

_____

_____

_____

Action Steps

- ESSENTIAL 5 ACTION: There is a saying that goes, "If you want something done, give it to a busy person." We have changed that to, "If you want something done well, give it to a busy, successful person." Busy, *successful* people have learned how to compartmentalize their time so that they can get *multiple* things done better than many people can get one thing done. They are able to focus. Focus in a war means you can't be looking at or thinking about something else. Your total energies are centered on the battle at hand. Being distracted can be the difference between success and failure, life or death. When you're putting time into an area of your life, it also needs focused energy. We call this present time consciousness or up time (UT). (See more about up time in chapter 7, "Essential 5: Maximize Peace and Strong Relationships.")

Now get busy on maximizing your lives by listing them all:

My Lives

1. _____

2. _____

3. _____

4. _____

5. _____

6. _____

7. _____

8. _____

9. _____

10. _____

Now that you can see your many lives listed, you can begin to prioritize how you spend time living them.

- ESSENTIAL 5 ACTION: Write out your To-do list, including how you'll serve your many lives, and add it to your war plan. IMPORTANT: Remember that Maximized Living is not about trying to squeeze so much into a day that your schedule is now jammed with To-dos. It's about having a plan, a framework, to make sure that you do not neglect what's important. When you have a war plan, all of your lives can flourish.

Don't forget to put the Big Four into your weekly war plan: shop, cook, prepare, plan. You'll never eat well without them.

- ESSENTIAL 5 ACTION: Create solid yellow boxes in your war plan that contain which day you will accomplish what items on the To-do list. Include what time you will start to accomplish it and how much time you will designate for this event or task. Each life will not go in each day. Some lives may not even go in each week. Enough quantity and quality time should be invested in each life in direct proportion to how important that particular life is and the need to be effective in it.

Reminder: PRIORITIZE, PRIORITIZE, PRIORITIZE! Make sure that date nights with your family and your fitness times are placed in solid yellow boxes.

- ESSENTIAL 5 ACTION: Timelessness—Write down how living in up time (UT) has allowed you to live without worry of upcoming tasks.
- ESSENTIAL 3 ACTION: Keep following the Intermediate Max Diet. Continue to eliminate sugars/carbohydrates after 3:00 p.m. Manage any cravings with the stay full and multiple feedings rules.
- ESSENTIAL 3 ACTION: Continue following the addition rule. Eat one Max food at breakfast, two at midday, and two in the late afternoon and evening.
- ESSENTIAL 3 ACTION: Keep taking your multivitamin with minerals.
- ESSENTIAL 4 ACTION: Do your SURGE.
- ESSENTIAL 5 ACTION: Continue the Peace Triathlon.

Elite Makeover Challenge

Day 8:

Exercise: Build Your Muscles

Weight training is the key to building muscle. The more muscle gained, the more fat lost. Also, the better your body ratio of muscle to fat is, the longer you will live. Weight training is an essential component to your exercise program, in addition to your cardiovascular SURGES.

Action Steps

Continue all your action steps from the Intermediate Makeover Challenge.

- ESSENTIAL 5 ACTION: Meditate during your Peace Triathlon.
- ESSENTIAL 5 ACTION: Put on your attitude of gratitude.
- ESSENTIAL 1 AND 3 ACTION: Check your pH balance and eat alkaline foods.
- ESSENTIAL 3 ACTION: Continue to follow the Intermediate or Elite Advanced Healing Diet.
- ESSENTIAL 4 ACTION: Begin your SURGE training for the week.
- ESSENTIAL 4 ACTION: Pause Sets. Keep a daily log of the weights you are using for each exercise and begin weekly increases of three percent. For example, if you bench pressed 100 pounds this first week, you will bench press 103 pounds the second week.

Intermediate Makeover Challenge

Day 9

Man-foods and the "Replacement Rule"

Man-foods are foods that are created, packaged and processed by man rather than grown or raised to eat. What you need to know about man-foods is that they are almost all indigestible. These are also foods that were not designed for the express purpose of being consumed or processed by your body on a regular basis. The farther away you get from eating the foods that are specifically created for your body, or the farther away these foods are from their natural form, the less efficiently the digestive system can break them down—if it all.

The bottom line is that man-food just sits there. Because these foods cannot pass through the digestive system quickly and cannot be broken down well, they will linger inside your body.

Maximized Living Number-One Nutrition Rule:

The farther away any product is from its natural state, the more potentially harmful it is to your body. Therefore, these foods are highly likely to poison and damage your body and should definitely be considered "harmful if swallowed."

For example: aspartame, fast-food burgers and fries, sugar, dairy products like milk, cheese, and ice cream, and refined flour products like breads, pastries, and cereal. These are all foods that are far removed from their natural states.

The Replacement Rule

No one will find it easy to give up all of their sweets, breads, fast-foods, and processed foods at once. In fact, we promised you that the Maximized Living Makeover challenges were about adding, not eliminating, foods from your diet. However, by adding enough good or Max foods to your diet, you will naturally eliminate or cut down on the amount of bad foods (man-foods) you consume. Look for healthier versions of your favorite bad foods so that you can begin to replace the worst of these foods with healthier alternatives.

Examples of the Replacement Rule

MAN-FOOD	REPLACEMENT
Pizza	Whole-grain pizza with all-natural sauce and low-fat, unrefined cheese.
Ice cream	Organic, low-fat alternative
Sugary, refined cereal	One of the many health-food, whole-grain cereals
Sugar	Honey, fresh fruit juice, unrefined maple syrup, molasses, brown rice syrup
Salt, MSG	Healthy spices and condiments
Rich desserts	Whole-grain, nondairy, chemical-free, low-fat, or honey- or fruit-sweetened treats
Fast-food burger	Grass-fed, all-beef burger; free-range turkey burger; or veggie burger
Cheese	Raw or goat cheese

Be creative when using the replacement rule. What man-foods can you replace with healthier or health food store alternatives?

Action Steps

- ESSENTIAL 3 ACTION: Follow the Intermediate Max Diet.
- ESSENTIAL 3 ACTION: Remember the addition rule. Add Max foods; don't eliminate. Eliminating will be the natural result of adding. Eat five or more Max foods a day with only eating vegetables, proteins, and fats after 3:00 p.m.
- ESSENTIAL 3 ACTION: Keep taking your multivitamin with minerals. Add an omega-3 fatty acid supplement each day.
- ESSENTIAL 3 ACTION: Begin to replace some of the most potent man-foods with natural alternatives. This is the replacement rule.
- ESSENTIAL 3 ACTION: Continue the multiple-feedings rule: Eat at least three times a day, with four to five times a day really being the best.
- ESSENTIAL 3 ACTION: Follow the stay-full rule: Eat enough Max foods a day to prevent cravings.
- ESSENTIAL 3 ACTION: Remember the Big Four: Keep planning, preparing, cooking, and shopping in your daily and weekly schedule.
- ESSENTIAL 4 ACTION: Do your SURGE
- ESSENTIAL 5 ACTION: Continue your Peace Triathlon.
- ESSENTIAL 5 ACTION: Continue to work your war plan. If you fail to plan, you plan to fail.

Elite Makeover Challenge

Day 9
Pound the H_2O

Water is the most important nutrient for your body. Water is needed for every function and process in your body. You lose up to two quarts of water per day, and if you don't replenish it you will become dehydrated. Dehydration is responsible for many health issues and symptoms.

Action Steps

Continue all your action steps from the Intermediate Makeover Challenge.
- Essential 1 and 3 action: Check your pH balance and eat alkaline foods.
- Essential 3 action: Continue to follow the Intermediate or Elite Max Diet.
- Essential 1 and 3 action: Begin drinking at least one-half quart of water (16 oz.) daily for every fifty pounds of body weight.

Start drinking greens powders in your water to help alkalize the water and give you the detoxifying benefits of greens.

Make sure you have a good water filter. Ideally, you should have one that even puts water at the correct pH. Another option is to add pH drops to your water. You can learn about filters and green powders at www.MaximizedLivingMakeover.com.
- •Essential 4 action: Continue your SURGE training.
- •Essential 5 action: Put on your attitude of gratitude.
- •Essential 5 action: Meditate during your Peace Triathlon.

Intermediate Makeover Challenge

Day 10
The Truth About Training: Take a "Pause"

Let's look at some of the myths surrounding fitness training, moving your body, or what is commonly called "exercise." What is the real truth? Is making yourself sweat really good for you? Let's take a look:

Myth: Exercising hurts.

Truth: Healthy movement is comfortable and can help to prevent, not cause, pain.

⚡Myth: Exercise takes hours, and you have to work out every day to get or stay in shape.

⚡Note: It takes literally three minutes to complete a Pause Set.

Now that you know the truth about exercise, it's time to take your SURGEs and crank them up a notch. We're going to add Pause Sets, with the goal of working out each part of the body each week.

Pause Sets equal one specific exercise each for chest, biceps, triceps, and abdominal muscles (abs) or one specific exercise each for legs (squats or lunges), calves, shoulders, and back/lateral muscles (lats). Each exercise takes only three minutes, for a total of ten to twelve minutes of exercise and can be done in between SURGE days or added to a SURGE day if it fits better into your schedule to do all of your exercising in one day. For example, add a Pause Set on day 11 and day 13 before your SURGE and take day 10 and day 12 off from exercise.

Action Steps

- ESSENTIAL 4 ACTION: Add Pause Sets this week. The goal is to hit each body part each week. Pause Sets: Do one exercise each for chest, biceps, triceps, and abs. Each exercise takes only three minutes for a total of ten to twelve minutes of exercise. (You can also move this to a SURGE day if it fits better into the schedule for you to get all your exercise done on one day and get an extra day off from exercise. For example, do this on day 11 and day 13 before your SURGE and take day 10 and day 12 off from exercise.)
- ESSENTIAL 5 ACTION: Follow your war plan.
- ESSENTIAL 3 ACTION: Intermediate Max Diet. Continue to eliminate sugars/carbohydrates after 3:00 p.m. Manage any cravings with the stay-full and multiple-feedings rules.
- ESSENTIAL 3 ACTION: Continue following the addition rule. Eat one Max-food at breakfast, two at midday, and two in the late afternoon and evening.
- ESSENTIAL 3 ACTION: Keep taking your multivitamin with minerals and omega-3 supplements.
- ESSENTIAL 5 ACTION: Continue the Peace Triathlon.

Elite Makeover Challenge

Day 10

Feel the Need for Speed

Now that you have been doing SURGE training for a while (especially if you completed the Intermediate Makeover Challenge), it's time to pick up the pace. For the Elite Makeover Challenge, you need to push your body a little harder by increasing the speed at which you SURGE.

Action Steps

Continue all your action steps from the Intermediate Makeover Challenge.

- ESSENTIAL 1 AND 3 ACTION: Check your pH balance, eat alkaline foods, drink greens daily.
- ESSENTIAL 1 AND 3 ACTION: Drink at least one-half quart (16 oz.) of water for every fifty pounds of body weight, add pH drops and use an alkalizing filter.
- ESSENTIAL 3 ACTION: Continue to follow the Intermediate or Elite/Advanced Healing Max Diet.
- ESSENTIAL 4 ACTION: During cardio/SURGE training, increase your speed gradually this week and each of the following weeks. Set a goal, and gradually increase until you reach it. For example: Your goal may be to increase output by surging from ten seconds to twenty seconds.
- ESSENTIAL 4 ACTION: Pause as a Monster Set. A Monster Set is when, instead of resting after performing an exercise on one body part, you immediately perform an exercise on *another* body part. The other body part should be one that was not used while exercising the first body part. For example: combine chest and biceps, or quadriceps and hamstrings.
- ESSENTIAL 5 ACTION: Put on your attitude of gratitude.
- ESSENTIAL 5 ACTION: Meditate during your Peace Triathlon.

Intermediate Makeover Challenge

Day 11
Become Want-less

Telling you not to want anything is some exceptionally good advice. Unfortunately, wanting is human nature. You were literally born wanting. When wanting becomes a problem is when you go from just wanting food and a dry diaper to wanting a nicer car, a bigger home, a different job, a better body, a larger bank account, a tropical vacation, and the latest electronic gadget. As you begin to desire more and more, what you desire begins to drive your thoughts, control your actions, and determine the direction you and your emotions go.

When your personal litmus test of how well you are doing is based on how many of your wants you have actually achieved or are close to getting, you have become a slave to your wants. Ultimately, your wants become your masters.

To continue to create peace and fulfill essential 5, you must learn to become both ambitious and content. Yes, you should set goals and always strive to achieve more, but be happy with what you already possess. Have wants, but also be *want-less*. You don't "want" your way into peace of mind.

Constantly seeking more will often cause you to look past what is truly important. If you believe you must reach your goals to be worthy or satisfied with life, you will rarely, if ever, find peace. Being a miserable achiever is practically a proverb. Perhaps the most universal thing people think they want is financial freedom, because they believe that money will bring them peace. The problem is, there is no such thing as financial freedom. If you do not have money, you worry about where you are going to get it. If you have it, you worry about it being taken away. The bottom line is, if you want money, you are going to worry about money.

Like money, the tragedy of getting what you want is that it never really ends up being truly fulfilling, and it almost never satisfies the want. Cars get old, gadgets get broken, and vacations end. Acquisitions rarely bring lasting joy and usually bring with them even more concern about money.

As you begin the action steps for day 11, focus on becoming want-less.

Action Steps
- ESSENTIAL 3 ACTION: Continue the Intermediate Max Diet. Continue eliminating the toxic man-foods from your diet using the Replacement Rule while looking to save the ones you really crave for vacation day—day 14.
- ESSENTIAL 3 ACTION: Continue the addition rule: Eat five or more Max foods a day, only eating vegetables, proteins, and fats after 3:00 p.m.

- ESSENTIAL 3 ACTION: Continue the multiple-feedings rule: Eat at least three times a day, with four to five times a day really being the best.
- ESSENTIAL 3 ACTION: Follow the stay-full rule: Eat enough Max foods a day to prevent getting hungry.
- ESSENTIAL 3 ACTION: Remember the Big Four: Keep planning, preparing, cooking, and shopping in your daily and weekly schedule.
- ESSENTIAL 3 ACTION: Keep taking your multivitamin with minerals and your omega-3 fats. Other good basic supplements: Greens powder in your water and Grass-fed whey protein shake.
- ESSENTIAL 4 ACTION: Do Your SURGE.
- ESSENTIAL 5 ACTION: Continue the Peace Triathlon.
- ESSENTIAL 5 ACTION: Follow your war plan.
- ESSENTIAL 5 ACTION: Be want-less.

Elite Makeover Challenge

Day 11

Breakfast: The Most Important Meal of the Day

We've all heard again and again (in lots of sugary cereal television commercials) that breakfast is the most important meal of the day. Well, that's absolutely true! It's just common sense. Your body just went without food as you slept for at least eight hours. You "fasted" during the hours you slept. Now it's time to "break" the "fast." That's breakfast, the breaking of the fast.

Because it's the most important meal, it also needs to be a very nutritious meal so that you can jumpstart your day. One good way to get the nutrients you need is to start each morning with the most nutritious shake you can make. A morning shake is the quickest way to get the vitamins, minerals, antioxidants, and protein into your body. It is also the easiest for your body to digest.

Action Steps

Continue all your action steps from the Intermediate Makeover Challenge.
- ESSENTIAL 1 AND 3 ACTION: Check your pH balance, eat alkaline foods, and drink greens daily.
- ESSENTIAL 1 AND 3 ACTION: Drink at least one-half quart (16 oz.) of water for every fifty pounds of body weight, add pH drops, and use an alkalizing filter.

- ESSENTIAL 3 ACTION: Continue to follow the Intermediate or Elite "Advanced Healing" Diet.
- ESSENTIAL 3 ACTION: Grass-fed whey smoothie: Start the morning with a nutritious shake. Here is an example: 1 cup of coconut milk, ½ cup water, fresh blueberries, raspberries, strawberries, 2 scoops of unpasteurized whey protein, ice. Mix these ingredients in a blender and drink.
- ESSENTIAL 4 ACTION: During cardio/SURGE training, increase your speed gradually this week.
- ESSENTIAL 5 ACTION: Put on your attitude of gratitude.
- ESSENTIAL 5 ACTION: Meditate during your Peace Triathlon.

Intermediate Makeover Challenge

Day 12
Winning the Battle and the War

How are you doing on your war plan? Are you sticking to it? Each To-do you accomplish, every date time you fulfill, every time you check off that you did your SURGE training, and every time you do something that builds some more "mental muscle," count it as a victory! Each To-do you accomplish is another battle won against the war on your family, your mind, and your body that so many are losing. Keep winning the battles, and you'll surely win the war.

It's time now to turn to Essentials 1 and 2. We've spent the first eleven days focusing around health (Essential 3), fitness (Essential 4) and the time and schedule management skills that promote mental, emotional, and relational well-being (Essential 5). But what about the other two? They are called Essentials because they are just as necessary to Maximized Living as the other three.

In order to begin focusing on Essential 1, it's time to answer the question: what are the poisons from the Toxic Top Ten in your life? Are they medications? If so, talk to your doctor about reducing or eliminating medicines because you're now getting healthy. If they won't help, find a new doctor! If household products are on your toxic list, make it a point today to research, ask friends about, or go buy some natural alternatives. (Vinegar works wonders when cleaning.) Are packaged, processed foods your major downfall? Read labels and avoid foods with chemicals, bad fats, preservatives, colorings, and sugars (Sugar or anything with "-ose" at the end, which is sugar in disguise, like fructose, lactose, etc.)

For Essential 2, it's time to get educated. You can't achieve maximized living unless you understand and believe that maximum nerve supply is essential to your overall health and well-being. Learn what you need to do to have maximum nerve supply.

There's no way to be healthy without it. Investigate chiropractors, looking for ones that can help you achieve a corrected, normal, healthy spine and nervous system. Also, you should schedule a set of spine x-rays to see if your spine is properly aligned. To learn how to find help, go to www.MaximizedLivingMakeover.com.

Action Steps

- ESSENTIAL 1 ACTION: Make a list of the Toxic Top Ten in your life and eliminate as many items as you can today. Get rid of toxic foods and household products and buy some natural alternatives. Make an appointment with your doctor to talk about reducing or eliminating medications.
- ESSENTIAL 2 ACTION: Look into chiropractors in your area. Ask friends and family who they would recommend. Quiz them about their results. Educate yourself on the importance of maximum nerve supply for your life. Schedule your spine x-rays.
- ESSENTIAL 3 ACTION: Continue the Intermediate Max Diet. Continue eliminating the toxic man-foods from your diet using the replacement rule while looking to save the ones you really crave for vacation day—day 14.
- ESSENTIAL 3 ACTION: Continue the addition rule: Eat five or more Max foods a day, only eating vegetables, proteins, and fats after 3:00 p.m.
- ESSENTIAL 3 ACTION: Continue the multiple-feedings rule: Eat at least three times a day, with four to five times a day really being the best.
- ESSENTIAL 3 ACTION: Follow the stay-full rule: Eat enough Max foods a day to prevent getting hungry.
- ESSENTIAL 3 ACTION: Remember the Big Four: Keep planning, preparing, cooking, and shopping in your daily and weekly schedule.
- ESSENTIAL 3 ACTION: Keep taking your multivitamin with minerals and your omega-3 fats. Other good basic supplements: Greens powder in your water and grass-fed whey protein shake.
- ESSENTIAL 4 ACTION: Do your Pause Sets: One exercise each for legs (squat or lunge), calves, shoulders, back/lats for ten to twelve minutes of exercise. (Remember, you can also move this to a SURGE day if it fits better into the schedule to get the exercise done on one day and get an extra day off. For example, you can do this before your SURGE on day 13 and take day 12 off of exercise.)
- ESSENTIAL 5 ACTION: Continue your Peace Triathlon.
- ESSENTIAL 5 ACTION: Write down the progress you've made in your war plan and how it has helped you have less stress, anxiety, and rush in your life.

Elite Makeover Challenge

Day 12

Dump the Drinks

Almost everything you drink is toxic and full of sugar. Soda, coffee, juices, Gatorade, and energy drinks are full of toxic chemicals and lots of sugar, all of which destroy your immune system. Water is the best beverage by far for your health.

However, tap water is full of toxins, chlorine, and other dangerous chemicals. Choose bottled water, reverse osmosis, or filtered water as the best water for your health.

Action Steps

Continue all your action steps from the Intermediate Makeover Challenge.

- ESSENTIAL 1 AND 3 ACTION: Check your pH balance and eat alkaline foods.
- ESSENTIAL 3 ACTION: Continue to follow the Intermediate or Elite /Advanced Healing Max Diet.
- ESSENTIAL 4 ACTION: Do your cardio/SURGE training.
- ESSENTIAL 4 ACTION: Pause with Monster Set training. Two to three exercises per body part.
- ESSENTIAL 5 ACTION: Put on your attitude of gratitude.
- ESSENTIAL 5 ACTION: Meditate during your Peace Triathlon.
- ESSENTIAL 3 ACTION: Begin switching from coffee, soda and juices to water. Drink your one-half quart of water for every fifty pounds of body weight, and try not to drink anything else.

Intermediate Makeover Challenge

Day 13

Make "Better" Your Favorite Word

When coaches, fathers, and employers try to motivate their players, children, or staff, they often say, "Give me 110 percent!" This is the modern American way of saying 100 percent just isn't good enough anymore. That's one of the reasons why most people's New Year's resolutions have already gone the way of eight-track tapes, record albums, and the hustle by January 4. The problem is that people have a hard time handling the major change they've heaped on themselves. It's just too much pressure.

If you're a smoker, you've probably tried to quit many times. If you aren't happy with your weight or your waist size, you've probably begun and quit multiple diets and exercise plans. Most likely, you have also attempted to be more positive, more outgoing, or struggled to make some other changes in your attitude and fallen short.

Why?

It's not just because you're weak or unmotivated or don't know the statistics for problems associated with not taking care of your body. It's because change is extremely difficult, especially when you've made failure not an option. And especially if you want the change to take place all at once—110 percent!

Instead, consider getting 1 percent better every day. Life is not a game of perfect. You can't be, give or do 110 percent. Life is a game of many, many, many mistakes. We're up, we're down, we're good, we're not so good. It's all part of the package. Head toward your goal of Maximized Living with your eyes open. You will mess up. We guarantee it. Yet if you can look back on the last week and say you're 7 percent better (1 percent better each day for the last seven days), then you're a success.

The point is to keep moving forward. It's not so important where you are right now. What matters is where you're headed. Just keep getting better. It only takes a few weeks of *better* to equal a makeover. So make *better* your favorite word, and lose the word *perfect*.

EVALUATE: Over the past twelve days, what's gotten better in your life? Even 1 percent better counts!

_____

_____

_____

_____

Action Steps

- ESSENTIAL 1 ACTION: Keep eliminating toxins.
- ESSENTIAL 3 ACTION: Continue to follow the Intermediate Max Diet.
- ESSENTIAL 3 ACTION: Continue the food replacement rule.
- ESSENTIAL 3 ACTION: Continue eliminating the toxic man-foods from your diet, looking to save the ones you really crave for vacation day—tomorrow!
- ESSENTIAL 3 ACTION: Continue the addition rule.
- ESSENTIAL 3 ACTION: Continue the multiple-feedings rule.
- ESSENTIAL 3 ACTION: Continue the stay-full rule.
- ESSENTIAL 3 ACTION: Remember the Big Four.
- ESSENTIAL 3 ACTION: Take your basic supplements (multivitamin, omega-3, greens powder, grass-fed whey protein).
- ESSENTIAL 4 ACTION: Do your SURGE (and your Pause Set, if you have moved all your exercise to the same days).
- ESSENTIAL 5 ACTION: Continue the Peace Triathlon.
- ESSENTIAL 5 ACTION: Follow your war plan.

Elite Makeover Challenge

Day 13

Eat the Right Proportions

Make sure that every meal you eat contains the right healthy proportions of carbohydrates, fats, and proteins. The key to the correct proportions is to aim to consume 40 percent, the majority, of your calories from the fresh fruit and vegetables carbohydrates rather than carbohydrates like flours, grains, breads, pastas, rice, potatoes, and sugar. Berries are the recommended fruit, and keep your fruit intake limited to the morning.

Eat 30 percent of your calories from the right kinds of fats, and eat the last 30 percent from proteins taken from items like organic chicken and turkey, grass-fed beef, and wild (not farm-raised) fish. You can revisit chapter 5 for a list of Max foods.

Make sure every meal is close to this ratio. Plan out your meals ahead of time to ensure you will accomplish this. One easy way to do this is to reverse your portions. Go from having a big bowl of pasta and tiny bowl of salad to a huge bowl of salad and tiny bowl of carbs. (Don't eat any pasta if you are following the Advanced Healing Max Diet.)

Remember that in the Advanced Healing Max Diet, reducing grains, flours, sugars, pasta, rice, and potatoes is the healthiest choice and will cause major positive changes in your health, your hormones, and your body type. If you're sick, detoxifying, or looking for a substantial change in lifestyle, weight and overall health, then keep following this program.

Action Steps

Continue all your action steps from the Intermediate Makeover Challenge.

- ESSENTIAL 1 AND 3 ACTION: Check your pH balance, eat alkaline foods, and drink greens daily.
- ESSENTIAL 1 AND 3 ACTION: Keep switching from coffee, soda, and juices to water. Drink your one-half quart of water, using an alkalizing filter for every fifty pounds of body weight, use pH drops, and try not to drink anything else.
- ESSENTIAL 3 ACTION: If you are following the Elite Max Diet, stick to it. If not, begin to eat fewer carbohydrates from flours, grains, breads, pastas, rice, potatoes, and sugar sources, and replace them with more vegetable carbs.
- ESSENTIAL 4 ACTION: Do your cardio/SURGE training and Pause Sets, if you're working weights into your SURGE day.
- ESSENTIAL 5 ACTION: Put on your attitude of gratitude.
- ESSENTIAL 5 ACTION: Meditate during your Peace Triathlon.

Intermediate Makeover Challenge

Day 14

Vacation Day—Wow!

It's the end of your second week of the Maximized Living Intermediate Makeover Challenge, and you're officially on vacation—but only for the day and only in the food category. Today is the day you can indulge—to a point. Vacation meals are made up of either healthy foods that are a break from the more traditional ways of the un-diet (like bread and pasta), or the real live junk foods you crave (like chocolate and pizza).

You don't "cheat" on our undiet. If you're overwhelmed by a craving, you make that a vacation meal, and you get back to the plan. It's not a cave when you crave with a plan in place. Maximized Living is a lifetime lifestyle.

Action Steps

- ESSENTIAL 1 ACTION: Keep eliminating toxins.
- ESSENTIAL 3 ACTION: Intermediate Max Diet.
- ESSENTIAL 3 ACTION: Take your vacation meal!
- ESSENTIAL 3 ACTION: Continue with the food replacement rule.
- ESSENTIAL 3 ACTION: Continue eliminating the toxic man-foods from your diet, looking to save the ones you really crave for vacation day (today and every seven days).

- ESSENTIAL 3 ACTION: Continue the addition rule.
- ESSENTIAL 3 ACTION: Continue the multiple-feedings rule.
- ESSENTIAL 3 ACTION: Continue the stay-full rule.
- ESSENTIAL 3 ACTION: Remember the Big Four.
- ESSENTIAL 3 ACTION: Take your supplements.
- ESSENTIAL 3 ACTION: Remember: Conscious eating. Stay conscious of what you put in your body!
- ESSENTIAL 5 ACTION: Write out your To-do list for week 3.
- ESSENTIAL 5 ACTION: Remember to keep your priorities in order and put nonnegotiables like family times in solid yellow boxes.

Diets like the Max Intermediate Diet require additional shopping and some online shopping. Go to www.MaximizedLivingMakeover.com or on-line shopping advice, shopping lists, and meal plans.

Elite Makeover Challenge

Day 14

Assess Yourself: The Weekly Update

Can you believe it? Two weeks have already flown by, and you are well on your way to achieving your goal of Maximized Living. You are making improvements daily in the quality of your eating, exercise habits, and state of mind. Now let's see how far you've come from last week. Assess your life, your daily habits, your nutrition, your exercise and look to see how much you improved. You may not think you've changed that much until you look back at where you were.

Take your measurements and answer the following questions again:

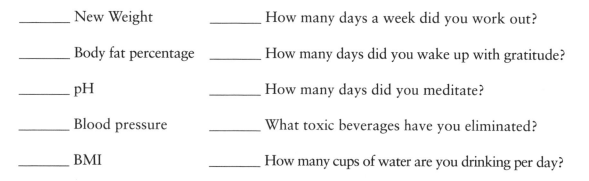

_____ New Weight	_____ How many days a week did you work out?
_____ Body fat percentage	_____ How many days did you wake up with gratitude?
_____ pH	_____ How many days did you meditate?
_____ Blood pressure	_____ What toxic beverages have you eliminated?
_____ BMI	_____ How many cups of water are you drinking per day?

Action Steps

Continue all your action steps from the Intermediate Makeover Challenge.

- ESSENTIAL 1 AND 3 ACTION: Drink at least one-half quart (16 oz.) of water for every fifty pounds of body weight, add pH drops, and use an alkalizing filter.
- ESSENTIAL 1 AND 3 ACTION: Check your pH balance, eat alkaline foods, and drink greens daily.
- ESSENTIAL 2 ACTION: Make sure you are staying on track with your chiropractic adjustments and at home spinal exercises.
- ESSENTIAL 3 ACTION: Stick to the Elite Max Diet or eat fewer carbs and replace with more vegetables.
- ESSENTIAL 5 ACTION: Put on your attitude of gratitude.
- ESSENTIAL 5 ACTION: Meditate during your Peace Triathlon.

Intermediate Makeover Challenge

Day 15

Reminder of the Three Basic Changes and Max Foods List That Make Up the Beginner and Intermediate Max Diets

The Three Basic Changes

1. If you are eating man-made fats, simply replace them with good, non-man-made fats. (See Max foods Good Fats List in chapter five.)
2. If you are eating man-made meats, simply replace them with good, non-man-made fats and meats. Order better meats to eat as often as fits into your budget. Remember, we call this a very good investment because it's your health and your future.
3. Take a stricter approach to eliminating sugar and processed grains, particularly in the afternoons and evenings. You will look and feel so much better!

Here is a little sentence to help you remember the Three Basic Changes.
Just think **"MEET FAT SALLY."**

1. **Meet:** Change to grass-fed max **meat** (And free-range chicken and eggs)!
2. **Fat:** Change from man **fats** to good Max **fats**!
3. **Sally:** Change to whole grains and remove all processed grains and **sugars**!

The Intermediate Max Diet limits grain intake to one meal a day from specific grains choices. It also limits your fruit intake to Max fruits. Refresh your memory by rereading about the Intermediate Max Diet in chapter 5 or simply go to www.MaximizedLivingMakeover.com.

Action Steps

- ESSENTIAL 3 ACTION: Continue eliminating the toxic man-foods from your diet using the replacement rule.
- ESSENTIAL 3 ACTION: Continue the addition rule. Eat five or more Max foods a day, eating only vegetables, proteins, and fats after 3:00 p.m.
- ESSENTIAL 3 ACTION: Continue the multiple-feedings rule: Eat at least three times a day, with four to five times a day really being the best.
- ESSENTIAL 3 ACTION: Follow the stay-full rule: Eat enough Max foods a day to prevent cravings.
- ESSENTIAL 3 ACTION: Remember the Big Four: Keep planning, preparing, cooking, and shopping in your daily and weekly schedule.
- ESSENTIAL 3 ACTION: Take your multivitamin with minerals.
- ESSENTIAL 4 ACTION: Do your SURGE.
- ESSENTIAL 5 ACTION: Stay on the war path with your war plan. At this point, you should feel good about not missing dates with family, workouts, or getting stuck without the proper foods in the house, at work, or during meetings and travel.
- ESSENTIAL 5 ACTION: Continue your Peace Triathlon.

Elite Makeover Challenge

Day 15

Seek Professional Supplement Advice

The best source of nutrients for our bodies is food. However, our foods no longer have the same amount of nutrients that they did when we were younger. Today, it is crucial to do the basics in order to help your body get the nutrients it needs to work.

The basic supplement regime you've been following supplements your diet daily with a high-quality multivitamin with minerals daily, along with a good greens powder and an omega-3 fatty acid product. For you, the Elite Makeover Challenge participant, you can go deeper into figuring out your personal supplement needs.

Outside of the basics, guessing at your specific needs can do more harm than good and will more than likely cost you extra money (and give you some pretty expensive urine as your body eliminates most of what you put in!). Refer back to chapter 5 for a good overview on how to get a legitimate nutritional assessment. Professional advice is a step above guessing, but you really need a qualified doctor trained in nutritional assessments. You can find one near you at www.MaximizedLivingMakeover.com.

Action Steps

Continue all your action steps from the Intermediate Makeover Challenge.

- ESSENTIAL 1 AND 3 ACTION: Check your pH balance, eat alkaline foods, and drink greens daily.
- ESSENTIAL 3 ACTION: Keep switching from coffee, soda and juices to water. Drink your one-half quart of water, using an alkalizing filter for every fifty pounds of body weight, use pH drops and try not to drink anything else.
- ESSENTIAL 3 ACTION: Stick to the Elite Max Diet or eat fewer carbs and replace with more vegetables.
- ESSENTIAL 3 ACTION: Find out from a pro if you have additional supplement requirements.
- ESSENTIAL 4 ACTION: Do your SURGE and Pause Set weight training with Monster Sets.
- ESSENTIAL 5 ACTION: Put on your attitude of gratitude.
- ESSENTIAL 5 ACTION: Meditate during your Peace Triathlon.

Intermediate Makeover Challenge

Day 16

Change Your Perceptions and Develop Your UTP

Each person on this planet was created with a unique design and a one-of-a-kind purpose to fulfill. Out of the billions of people on Earth, you will be the only one to live your exact life and carry out your life's mission—or not. But it's difficult to remember that you are unique and have great talents and skills. Life can beat the creativity right out of you sometimes. What you need is a fresh perspective and a change in your perceptions of yourself.

In order to fulfill your purpose, you need to know what your strength, skills, and talents are. What are you naturally really good at? What are you passionate about? If money wasn't an object and you could not fail, what would you be doing right now? Once you have answered these questions, you will have determined your Unique Talent Proposition (UTP).

Once you know your UTP, you can examine your life to see if you are playing to your strengths. Here's what we mean: The mistake people make in assessing Olympians and top pro athletes is that they see the athletes as extra strong, fast, technically superior, and flexible. People see them as having great balance, lightning quick reflexes, and more. The truth is, they usually don't have all these things. But they do have a couple of them.

What makes most great athletes great and, in fact, it's the same thing that makes most of the great people throughout history great, is not that they had a dozen talents.

What they usually have is just one great talent that they totally capitalized on. They took one great attribute and worked it and worked it until it became so immensely polished and powerful that it took them to the top.

Every person is better than a thousand other people at something. Yet if you never discover or develop your talent or talents, the gifts will be wasted. You possess very special and unique gifts. You have skills. These skills or talents may be hidden within you, so you must focus your life on finding them. They are your destiny.

You are incredibly valuable. You have gifts that will help meet the world's needs. You have an obligation to realize your potential. In the ideal world, everybody fully expresses their gifts in a way that helps the world. When you are using your gifts to fulfill whatever purpose and mission you have been given, you will find yourself feeling worthy and exceedingly effective, healthy, joyful, and at peace.

In order to truly understand your worth, you need to take four steps to changing your perception of yourself. Write your answers to the following questions and statements below:

1. Explain what you think your value is:

_____

_____

_____

_____

2. What is your unique talent proposition (UTP)?

_____

_____

_____

3. What is your higher purpose? How will you use your value and UTP to serve others, make a difference, and leave an impact on the world?

_____

_____

_____

_____

4. What are some values you will now live by based on your higher purpose? How will the rules change if you live for a cause vs. living for yourself?

_____

_____

_____

_____

Once you have focused on this process of self-examination, you will be able to see whether your time is being spent in the areas you were created to pursue. And you will know whether your goals and tasks center around yourself or are designed to benefit others.

⚡Note: Your value system is a protection against negative outside opinions and deferred results. Serve the mission, not the results, and let the rest sort itself out.

Action Steps
- ESSENTIAL 3 ACTION: Intermediate Max Diet
- ESSENTIAL 3 ACTION: Continue eliminating the toxic man-foods from your diet using the replacement rule while looking to save the ones you really crave for vacation day—day 21.
- ESSENTIAL 3 ACTION: Continue the addition rule: Eat five or more Max foods a day with only eating vegetables, proteins, and fats after 3:00 p.m.
- ESSENTIAL 3 ACTION: Continue the multiple-feedings rule: Eat at least three times a day, with four to five times a day really being the best.
- ESSENTIAL 3 ACTION: Follow the stay-full rule: Eat enough Max foods a day to prevent getting too hungry.
- ESSENTIAL 3 ACTION: Remember the Big Four: Keep planning, preparing, cooking, and shopping in your daily and weekly schedule.
- ESSENTIAL 3 ACTION: Take your multivitamin with minerals.
- ESSENTIAL 4 ACTION: Do your SURGE.
- ESSENTIAL 5 ACTION: Think about your value and worth, then figure out if you are spending yourself wisely.
- ESSENTIAL 5 ACTION: Continue daily Peace Triathlon.
- ESSENTIAL 5 ACTION: Continue to follow your war plan for today, and make sure you're prepared to work today's steps you took in changing perceptions into tomorrow's new war plan.

Elite Makeover Challenge

Day 16

Sleep. Enough Said.

Sleep is one of life's necessities. In April 2007, the Institute of Medicine issued a report that confirmed definite links between sleep deprivation and increased risks of hypertension, diabetes, obesity, depression, heart attack and stroke. A minimum of eight hours in total darkness every night is the appropriate amount of sleep for the average person.

Action Steps

Continue all your action steps from the Intermediate Makeover Challenge.

- ESSENTIAL 1 AND 3 ACTION: Check your pH balance, eat alkaline foods, and drink greens daily.
- ESSENTIAL 3 ACTION: Keep switching from coffee, soda and juices to water. Drink your one-half quart of water, using an alkalizing filter for every fifty pounds of body weight, use pH drops and try not to drink anything else.
- ESSENTIAL 3 ACTION: Stick to the Elite Max Diet or eat fewer carbs and replace with more vegetables.
- ESSENTIAL 3 ACTION: Take your multivitamin and mineral supplement.
- ESSENTIAL 4 ACTION: Do your SURGE/Pause Set training with Monster Sets.
- ESSENTIAL 5 ACTION: Begin tonight to go to bed earlier, in total darkness and with no television. Try to get eight hours or more sleep every night.
- ESSENTIAL 5 ACTION: Put on your attitude of gratitude.
- ESSENTIAL 5 ACTION: Meditate during your Peace Triathlon.

Intermediate Makeover Challenge

Day 17

The Toxic Top Ten Elimination Plan

As mentioned, you should be in the process of eliminating as many toxic chemicals, medications, and foreign products that your body comes in contact with as possible. Some of the places these are found may surprise you. Household cleaners are obvious, but have you ever stopped to check the labels on your toothpaste and deodorant? Have you examined your cookware? What about the air you breathe and water you drink? Are these life-giving substances as pure as you can get them?

Here are some ways you can follow essential 1 and create a plan to eliminate or reduce more toxins:

- MEDICATIONS: Your doctor should be helping you get off drugs that aren't absolutely keeping you alive. As you get healthier, you need a whole lot less drugs. Hopefully, none.
- AMALGAM FILLINGS: Do you have silver fillings? If so, you may be mercury toxic. To learn more, visit www.MaximizedLivingMakeover.com.
- HOUSEHOLD PRODUCTS: Start buying all-natural toothpaste. You swallow the stuff twice a day!
- COOKWARE: Look anywhere; all data points to the fact that Teflon is toxic. Switch to stainless steel, using good fats like extra virgin olive oil and cooking over low heat. Use raw butter and coconut oil to cook at higher heats.
- AIR AND WATER: For these two fairly important items, consider air and water purifiers.

For more help replacing the toxins in your life, visit MaximizedLivingMakeover.com.

Action Steps

- ESSENTIAL 1 ACTION: Eliminate as many toxins as possible from your daily routine.
- ESSENTIAL 3 ACTION: Continue to follow the Intermediate Max Diet.
- ESSENTIAL 3 ACTION: Continue food replacement rule. Eliminate the toxic man-foods from your diet, looking to save the ones you really crave for vacation day—day 21.
- ESSENTIAL 3 ACTION: Continue the addition rule. Eat five or more Max foods a day, only eating vegetables, proteins, and fats after 3:00 p.m.
- ESSENTIAL 3 ACTION: Continue the multiple-feedings rule.
- ESSENTIAL 3 ACTION: Continue the stay-full rule.
- ESSENTIAL 3 ACTION: Remember the Big Four.
- ESSENTIAL 3 ACTION: Take your supplements.
- ESSENTIAL 4 ACTION: Do Pause Sets for chest, biceps, triceps, and abs for a total of ten to twelve minutes of exercise (or move this to a SURGE day). If you are feeling ambitious, you can add an additional exercise (two instead of one) for all or just some of your tougher body parts.
- ESSENTIAL 5 ACTION: Continue your Peace Triathlon.
- ESSENTIAL 5 ACTION: Keep following your war plan.

Elite Makeover Challenge

Day 17

Tone Down Your Toxicity

When the United States EPA did biopsy studies of chemicals found in the fat of human beings, it showed 100 percent—every one—of the people studied had cancer-causing chemicals in their bodies! Toxicity is a major contributor to obesity and disease. You need to make it your goal to continue to tone down your toxicity.

If you're toxic, you may not be able to lose weight! It also will cause you to age rapidly, experience radically reduced libido, and/or live with degenerative illness, serious pain, and overt fatigue.

One area you may not have thought of that is responsible for introducing toxic chemicals to your body on a daily basis is your personal hygiene products. The products you put directly on your skin are being absorbed into your bloodstream. These include hand soaps, shampoos, lotions, toothpaste, makeup, deodorants, perfumes and colognes.

You have to be checked and cleansed! While step one is reducing exposure, you also have to detox. You can find helpful tips at www.MaximizedLivingMakeover.com. Additionally, there are a number of tests that are recommended for mercury, lead, and other heavy metals, as well as for bio-toxins due to molds and Lyme.

Action Steps

Continue all your action steps from the Intermediate Makeover Challenge. Sleep in total darkness for at least eight hours.

- ESSENTIAL 1 AND 3 ACTION: Check your pH balance, eat alkaline foods, and drink greens daily.
- ESSENTIAL 1 ACTION: Begin today to change over any product you put directly on your skin to more organic/natural/toxin-free products.
- ESSENTIAL 3 ACTION: Keep switching from coffee, soda and juices to water. Drink your one-half quart of water, using an alkalizing filter for every fifty pounds of body weight, use pH drops and try not to drink anything else.
- ESSENTIAL 3 ACTION: Stick to the Elite Max Diet or eat fewer carbs and replace with more vegetables.
- ESSENTIAL 3 ACTION: Take your supplements.
- ESSENTIAL 4 ACTION: Do your SURGE and/or weight training.
- ESSENTIAL 5 ACTION: Put on your attitude of gratitude.
- ESSENTIAL 5 ACTION: Meditate during your Peace Triathlon.

Intermediate Makeover Challenge

Day 18

Maximize Nerve Supply: Keep Your Power On!

As we've stated to you throughout this book, everything in your body– and that includes heart function, breathing, digestion, muscular development, fat-burning, and more— is under total control of the spine and nervous system. Think about it. You can go a month without food, days without water, and minutes without oxygen, but if you shut off the nerve supply, it's instant death. Life flows through the spine and nerves. If you cut a nerve to a cell, it's dead. Therefore, making a spinal evaluation part of your monthly pattern is not only important for wellness, it's essential for you to be fully alive.

Back in chapter 4, we discussed at length how crucial it is for your body to have maximum nerve supply at all times and how this can only be achieved through proper spinal care. Spinal care and maintenance can be performed by a chiropractor during your monthly visits, but it is also important for you to take good care of your spinal alignment in between chiropractic visits!

Posture plays a key role in this. Good posture keeps your power on. It keeps the nerve impulses flowing without blockages to all the parts of your body. Most of us have been told all our lives that we should "stand up straight," but good posture goes a lot further than that. So what does good posture really look like?

Stand in front of a full-length mirror to check your posture. Close your eyes and move your head up and down and side to side. Now open your eyes and check for the following: Is one shoulder higher than the other? Is your head turned or tilted to one side more than the other? Is your head in "computer posture" with your chin jutted out in front of your chest?

That's a quick home spine test to see if you are in alignment. If the answers to any of the above were yes, it's a good indication your power is off. Check with your chiropractor.

Learn everything you need to do to have maximum nerve supply. There's no way to express health without it. Investigate chiropractors looking for ones that can help you achieve a corrected, normal, healthy spine and nervous system. For more help, go to www.MaximizedLivingMakeover.com.

Action Steps

- ESSENTIAL 1 ACTION: Keep eliminating toxins.
- ESSENTIAL 2 ACTION: Evaluate your spinal health. How's your spine doing? Have tests revealed your nervous system has gotten better? Is your posture improved? If you still haven't made it to a chiropractor, make an appointment as soon as possible.

- ESSENTIAL 3 ACTION: Continue to follow the Max Intermediate Diet.
- ESSENTIAL 3 ACTION: Continue the food replacement rule.
- ESSENTIAL 3 ACTION: Continue eliminating the toxic man-foods from your diet, looking to save the ones you really crave for vacation day—day 21.
- ESSENTIAL 3 ACTION: Continue the addition rule.
- ESSENTIAL 3 ACTION: Continue the multiple-feedings rule.
- ESSENTIAL 3 ACTION: Continue the stay-full rule.
- ESSENTIAL 3 ACTION: Remember the Big Four.
- ESSENTIAL 3 ACTION: Remember, conscious eating. Stay conscious of what you put in your body!
- ESSENTIAL 3 ACTION: Take your supplements.
- ESSENTIAL 4 ACTION: Do your SURGE.
- ESSENTIAL 5 ACTION: Continue your Peace Triathlon.
- ESSENTIAL 5 ACTION: Work the war plan.

Elite Makeover Challenge

Day 18

Know Your EFA Ration

One of the most important healthy ratios in your body is your essential fatty acids (EFA) ratio. If your ratio is off, then you are building inflammation and disease in your body. The best way to protect yourself is to begin supplementing with fish oil or cod liver oil daily. If you know your diet is perfect and clean, then you will want to take flaxseed oil instead. There is specific testing that can be done to check this ratio with your Maximized Living doctor.

Omega-3 alert: omega-3s are part of the basic supplement recommendation. However, if you're eating a diet high in the good fats, then supplementing with omega-3 may actually create an imbalance. A fatty-acid ratio test can let you know if you need omega-3s, have too many omega-3s, or even need to supplement a different kind of fatty acid to restore balance.

Action Steps

Continue all your action steps from the Intermediate Makeover Challenge.
- ESSENTIAL 1 AND 3 ACTION: Check your pH balance, eat alkaline foods, and drink greens daily.
- ESSENTIAL 3 ACTION: Keep switching from coffee, soda and juices to water. Drink your one-half quart of water, using an alkalizing filter for every fifty pounds of body weight, use pH drops and try not to drink anything else.

- ESSENTIAL 3 ACTION: Stick to the Elite Max Diet or eat fewer carbs and replace with more vegetables.
- ESSENTIAL 3 ACTION: Take your supplements. Consult your Maximized Living doctor to see if your EFA ratio is off. If it is, begin taking the proper fatty acid based on these ratios.
- ESSENTIAL 4 ACTION: Do your SURGE/weight training. Continue to log your speeds or intensity for SURGE and your weights for your Pauses so that you're making sure to keep progressing!
- ESSENTIAL 5 ACTION: Put on your attitude of gratitude.
- ESSENTIAL 5 ACTION: Meditate during your Peace Triathlon.
- ESSENTIAL 5 ACTION: Sleep in total darkness for at least eight hours.

Intermediate Makeover Challenge

Day 19

Oxygen: The Most Important Nutrient

It's time to take a deeper look at what all this exercise is doing to change your body for the better. It all has to do with a little element called oxygen.

Here's why aerobic exercise is so important: Without it you are *choking to death* due to the fact that the body becomes depleted of oxygen and inefficient at taking it in, absorbing it, storing it, and using it. Common signs of oxygen depletion include:

- Fatigue
- Injury
- Memory loss
- Joint and muscle pain
- Infection
- Sleep disorder

- Low blood sugar
- Depression
- Problems Absorbing fat
- Decreased libido
- More difficult menstrual symptoms

Yikes! All of these health issues, simply because our bodies don't get enough life-giving, life-sustaining oxygen into each one of our cells. That should give you an extra incentive to do your SURGEs and Pause Sets to the max!

Action Steps

- ESSENTIAL 1 ACTION: Keep eliminating toxins.
- ESSENTIAL 3 ACTION: Keep sticking to the Max Three Basic Changes (Meet Fat Sally) and the Intermediate Max Diet.

- ESSENTIAL 3 ACTION: Continue all of the other nutrition changes (stay-full, replacement, multiple-feedings rules, etc.). Keep taking your supplements.
- ESSENTIAL 4 ACTION: Do your Pause Sets: one exercise each for legs (Squat or lunge), calves, shoulders, back/lats for ten to twelve minutes of exercise. (Remember, you can also move this to a SURGE day if it fits better into the schedule to get the exercise done on one day and get an extra day off.) You can also add an exercise for a body part that you want to move along faster. For example, if you have excess weight on the hips and thighs, you can throw in a lunge or a one-legged squat to help. Go to www.MaximizedLivingMakeover. com to find the right exercise for you and the proper way to do it.
- ESSENTIAL 5 ACTION: Plan the war plan; work the war plan.
- ESSENTIAL 5 ACTION: Continue your Peace Triathlon.

Elite Makeover Challenge

Day 19

Microwave Dangers

Continually eating food processed from a microwave oven causes long-term, permanent brain damage. Minerals, vitamins, and nutrients in all microwaved foods are reduced or altered so that the human body gets little or no benefit, or the human body absorbs altered compounds that cannot be broken down. The human body cannot metabolize (break down) the unknown by-products created in microwaved food.

Action Steps

Continue all your action steps from the Intermediate Makeover Challenge.
- ESSENTIAL 1 AND 3 ACTION: Check your pH balance, eat alkaline foods, and drink greens daily.
- ESSENTIAL 3 ACTION: Keep switching from coffee, soda and juices to water. Drink your one-half quart of water, using an alkalizing filter for every fifty pounds of body weight, use pH drops and try not to drink anything else.
- ESSENTIAL 3 ACTION: Stick to the Elite Max Diet or eat fewer carbs and replace with more vegetables.
- ESSENTIAL 3 ACTION: Take your recommended supplements.
- ESSENTIAL 1 ACTION: Continue to change over any product you put directly on your skin to more organic/natural/toxin-free products. From today on, stop using the microwave oven.
- ESSENTIAL 4 ACTION: Do your SURGE/weight training.

- ESSENTIAL 5 ACTION: Put on your attitude of gratitude.
- ESSENTIAL 5 ACTION: Meditate during your Peace Triathlon.
- ESSENTIAL 5 ACTION: Sleep in total darkness for at least eight hours.

Intermediate Makeover Challenge

Day 20

Finding Your Direction: Set Your "GPS."

As the third week of the Maximized Living Intermediate Makeover Challenge winds down, it is important to stop and evaluate whether or not you are headed in the right direction. You're making great progress in the areas of nutrition, fitness, spinal care, and eliminating toxins. You have learned to create To-do lists, fit them into a War Plan, and follow a schedule that frees up your life.

Now it's time to consider the big picture. Yes, it's great if you gas up the car properly, make sure it's in great running order, and get on the road. But if you don't have a destination in mind, you're just driving. So today it's time to add "GPS training" to your morning Peace Triathlon. (See chapter 7 if you need to brush up on this concept.) It's a process of self-evaluation to help you determine where you are going in life and if you are headed in the right direction to hit your destination.

1. Write down your three most important goals.

_____

_____

_____

_____

2. Write out your major goals in the present tense, as if they were already a reality.

_____

_____

_____

_____

3. Briefly describe what you are going to do today to achieve your goals. (Put these actions in a solid yellow box in your war plan.)

_____

_____

_____

_____

_____

4. Write your major problem or goal in the form of a question. For example, "How can I lose twenty-five pounds?" or "How can I be a more loving and caring spouse?" Write out your answers to this question.

_____

_____

_____

_____

_____

5. Select one action from the above exercise to begin immediately. (Also put this in a solid yellow box.)

_____

_____

_____

Using this exercise will help you work steadily toward the achievement of your goals throughout the day. You'll feel energized, hopeful, and powerful instead of fatigued, weak, and defeated. Remember, you must repeat this process every single day as part of your Peace Triathlon until it becomes a habit and is a permanent part of your brain's GPS circuitry.

Action Steps
- ESSENTIAL 5 ACTION: Add GPS Training to your Peace Triathlon.
- ESSENTIAL 1 ACTION: Keep eliminating toxins.
- ESSENTIAL 3 ACTION: Continue to follow the Intermediate Max Diet.

- ESSENTIAL 3 ACTION: Continue the food replacement rule.
- ESSENTIAL 3 ACTION: Continue eliminating the toxic man-foods from your diet, looking to save the ones you really crave for vacation day—day 21.
- ESSENTIAL 3 ACTION: Continue the addition rule.
- ESSENTIAL 3 ACTION: Continue the multiple-feedings rule.
- ESSENTIAL 3 ACTION: Continue the stay-full rule.
- ESSENTIAL 3 ACTION: Remember the Big Four.
- ESSENTIAL 3 ACTION: Remember, conscious eating. Stay conscious of what you put in your body!
- ESSENTIAL 3 ACTION: Keep taking your supplements.
- ESSENTIAL 4 ACTION: Do your SURGE.

Elite Makeover Challenge

Day 20
Tone Down Your Toxicity, Part 2

According to the EPA, our indoor environment is two to five times more toxic than our outdoor environment; and, in some cases, the air measurements indoors have been found to be one hundred times more polluted.[37] Most of the indoor pollution is caused from your household cleaning agents: oven cleaners, dishwashing detergent, laundry detergent, floor and furniture polishers, air fresheners, kitchen cleaners, carpet cleaners, and toilet bowl cleaners.

Tone down your toxicity by eliminating as many chemical-based cleaners as you can and replacing them with natural alternatives.

Action Steps
Continue all your action steps from the Intermediate Makeover Challenge.
- ESSENTIAL 5 ACTION: Put on your attitude of gratitude.
- ESSENTIAL 5 ACTION: Meditate during your Peace Triathlon.
- ESSENTIAL 5 ACTION: Sleep in total darkness for at least eight hours.
- ESSENTIAL 1 AND 3 ACTION: Check your pH balance, eat alkaline foods, and drink greens daily.
- ESSENTIAL 4 ACTION: Do your SURGE/weight training.
- ESSENTIAL 3 ACTION: Keep switching from coffee, soda and juices to water. Drink your one-half quart of water, using an alkalizing filter for every fifty pounds of body weight, use pH drops and try not to drink anything else.

- ESSENTIAL 3 ACTION: Stick to the Elite Max Diet or eat fewer carbs and replace with more vegetables.
- ESSENTIAL 3 ACTION: Take your recommended supplements.
- ESSENTIAL 1 ACTION: Continue to change over any product you put directly on your skin to more organic/natural/toxin-free products.
- ESSENTIAL 1 ACTION: Do not use the microwave oven.
- ESSENTIAL 1 ACTION: Begin today to switch from toxic cleaning products to natural, organic, or healthy products.

Intermediate Makeover Challenge

Day 21

Adjust Your War Plan

Congratulations! You've made it through three entire weeks of the Intermediate Makeover Challenge, and you should be feeling like a whole new you—or at least a 21 percent better you! As we enter the fourth week of the challenge, you should once again assess where you are now and how far you've come since you started on day 1.

As we prepare for the upcoming week, it is time to take an in-depth look at your war plan. War plans need continuous evaluation to determine if they are working—if they are taking you to your destination in the most efficient, healthy way. Here are a few of the warning signs or red flags that may pop up if your war plan is about to be derailed:

You Know You're in Trouble When...

- Your war plan isn't determining how you spend the week and days.
- You're not looking at the war plan before making time decisions.
- You have not updated the war plan. If you haven't, chances are good that people are losing out.
- You don't reset your war plan weekly to adapt to new items.
- You assume your GPS is set, or you have no time for Peace Triathlons. Rest assured, stress and negativity won't stop even if you stop preparing for it.

Your war plan is an essential component of your Peace Triathlon. Failing to be faithful to either or both can increase your stress level, decrease your health and destroy your peace of mind. And who wants that? No one! Be faithful to your morning Peace Triathlons, and update your war plan regularly to stay on track toward your goal of maximized living! (Oh yeah, and if you still feel the need to take one, it's vacation day. Enjoy foods you have been craving and the day off from exercise!)

Action Steps

- ESSENTIAL 1 ACTION: Keep eliminating toxins.
- ESSENTIAL 3 ACTION: Vacation day! If you still battle cravings, indulge them on this one day a week. Then, get back to your plan!
- ESSENTIAL 3 ACTION: Keep sticking to the Intermediate Max Diet.
- ESSENTIAL 3 ACTION: Continue all of the other nutrition changes (stay-full, replacement, and multiple-feedings rules, etc.).
- ESSENTIAL 3 ACTION: Keep taking your supplements.
- ESSENTIAL 5 ACTION: Update and evaluate your war plan. Make adjustments as necessary.
- ESSENTIAL 3 ACTION: Work the war plan.
- ESSENTIAL 3 ACTION: Peace Triathlon, including setting your GPS.

Elite Makeover Challenge

Day 21

Assess Yourself: The Weekly Update

Take your measurements, answer the familiar questions, and tally all the positive results you are seeing in many areas of your life. Congratulations on finishing week three of the Maximized Living Elite Makeover Challenge.

Take your measurements and answer the following questions again:

_____   New Weight

_____   Body fat percentage

_____   pH

_____   Blood pressure

_____   BMI

_____   How many days a week did you work out?

_____   How many days did you wake up with gratitude?

_____   How many days did you meditate?

_____   What toxic beverages have you eliminated?

_____   How many cups of water are you drinking per day?

_____   How many days are you doing your at-home spinal corrective exercises?

_____ Are you staying on track with your chiropractic adjustment schedule?

_____ How many days did you go without using microwave?

_____ How many household and personal cleaning products did you switch to natural?

_____ Has your pH improved?

_____ Are you taking all of your supplements?

_____ Have you had your EFA ratio tested?

Action Steps

Continue all your action steps from the Intermediate Makeover Challenge.

- ESSENTIAL 1 ACTION: Continue to change over any product you put directly on your skin to more organic/natural/toxin-free products.
- ESSENTIAL 1 ACTION: Keep replacing toxic, chemical-laden household cleaners with natural ones.
- ESSENTIAL 1 AND 3 ACTION: Check your pH balance, eat alkaline foods, and drink greens daily.
- ESSENTIAL 3 ACTION: Keep switching from coffee, soda and juices to water. Drink your one-half quart of water, using an alkalizing filter for every fifty pounds of body weight, use pH drops and try not to drink anything else.
- ESSENTIAL 3 ACTION: Stick to the Elite Max Diet or eat fewer carbs and replace with more vegetables.
- ESSENTIAL 3 ACTION: Take your recommended supplements.
- ESSENTIAL 3 ACTION: Keep eating a diet in the right proportions.
- ESSENTIAL 4 ACTION: Do your SURGE/weight training.
- ESSENTIAL 5 ACTION: Put on your attitude of gratitude.
- ESSENTIAL 5 ACTION: Meditate during your Peace Triathlon.
- ESSENTIAL 5 ACTION: Sleep in darkness for at least eight hours.

Intermediate Makeover Challenge

Day 22

Stay Clean

As you enter the fourth week of the Maximized Living Intermediate Challenge, your goals for maintaining the health of your body should be summed up by the phrase "stay clean"! Your body needs clean water, clean air, clean food, and clean (drug-free) blood.

Evaluate the progress you have made so far in replacing toxic personal hygiene products and household cleaners with natural/organic ones. Go check your refrigerator and pantry. Have you gotten rid of as many man-foods as possible and stocked up on fresh, living Max foods?

Have you consulted with your Maximized Living doctor about reducing and eventually eliminating any drugs your take, and are you staying active so that the oxygen can reach every cell in your body, helping it function at its peak? Make it your life motto as we head into these final days of the Maximized Living Intermediate Challenge—stay clean!

Action Steps

- ESSENTIAL 1 ACTION: Remember that toxins bind to fat cells, making looking and feeling good difficult. So stay clean—clean water, clean air, clean food, and clean (drug-free) blood.
- ESSENTIAL 2 ACTION: Keep your power on! Maintain good posture.
- ESSENTIAL 3 ACTION: Remember that continuing the addition rule, multiple-feeding rule, stay-full rule, and replacement rule will help you to Meet Fat Sally!
- ESSENTIAL 3 ACTION: Keep sticking to the Intermediate Max Diet.
- ESSENTIAL 3 ACTION: Keep taking your supplements.
- ESSENTIAL 4 ACTION: Do your SURGE.
- ESSENTIAL 5 ACTION: Plan the war plan; work the war plan.
- ESSENTIAL 5 ACTION: Continue Peace Triathlon, including setting your GPS.

Elite Makeover Challenge

Day 22
Clean from the Inside Out

Bowel movements are an important factor of your health. If you don't have at least one bowel movement per day, you are already heading down the path that leads to disease. Moving your bowels and keeping them clean starts with a diet in the right proportions: high in soluble vegetables and fruits (use the big bowl for these), fats and proteins (medium bowl), and whole grains in the small bowl only—or if you're doing the Elite/Advanced Healing Max Diet – not at all. Drinking water, eliminating toxins from your diet, reducing caffeine and alcohol (which are diuretics and cause dehydration), and radically lowering sugar intake are all critical to having a healthy colon.

A colon cleanse program is also incredibly helpful, and we hope you will get started on one today. Visit www.MaximizedLivingMakeover.com to learn more.

Action Steps

Continue all your action steps from the Intermediate Makeover Challenge.

- ESSENTIAL 1 ACTION: Continue to change over any product you put directly on your skin to more organic/natural/toxin-free products.
- ESSENTIAL 1 ACTION: Continue to use natural household cleaners.
- ESSENTIAL 1 ACTION: Begin a colon cleanse today.
- ESSENTIAL 1 AND 3 ACTION: Check your pH balance, eat alkaline foods, and drink greens daily.
- ESSENTIAL 3 ACTION: Keep switching from coffee, soda and juices to water. Drink your one-half quart of water, using an alkalizing filter for every fifty pounds of body weight, use pH drops and try not to drink anything else.
- ESSENTIAL 3 ACTION: Stick to the Elite Diet or eat fewer carbs and replace with more vegetables.
- ESSENTIAL 3 ACTION: Take your recommended supplements.
- ESSENTIAL 3 ACTION: Keep eating a diet in the right proportions.
- ESSENTIAL 4 ACTION: Do your SURGE/weight training. This week, start alternating Pause Sets with Decline Sets. Rather than using the same weight like you do for each Pause Set, lower the weight five to twenty pounds for each Decline Set. For example, if you do a Pause Set for your triceps, do a Decline Set for your biceps.
- ESSENTIAL 4 ACTION: Continue to do the body parts as a Monster set. NO REST between exercises. Rather then resting, alternate body parts. Now, you'll also be alternating between Pause Sets and Decline Sets.
- ESSENTIAL 5 ACTION: Put on your attitude of gratitude.
- ESSENTIAL 5 ACTION: Meditate during your Peace Triathlon.
- ESSENTIAL 5 ACTION: Sleep in darkness for at least eight hours.

Intermediate Makeover Challenge

Day 23

For Less Fat and More Health, You Must "Resist"

Due to the law of adaptation, muscles that are continuously under "resistance" become stronger, leaner, and better developed. The law of adaptation basically means that muscles will adapt to whatever force you apply to them—or don't. If you consistently put a strain on a certain muscle group, it will adapt by getting more physically powerful and more toned. It will change and improve its shape. If you consistently do not put strain on your muscles, they become weaker, flabbier, and shapeless.

Again, to be healthy, lean muscle mass must increase and fat must decrease. While aerobic exercises like walking or jogging will cause some resistance to the sets of muscles being used, they are not enough. Resistance needs to be applied throughout the entire body so that you remove fat and increase leanness in all or most of the muscles.

Resistance exercise occurs when you apply sustained or repetitive strain (resistance) to muscle. Resistance movements such as lifting weights and swimming have the potential to create strength gains, increase muscle tone, and decrease fat when done consistently and in the right manner. That's where your Pause Sets have been improving your overall workouts—by improving your muscle tone!

The Difference Between Men and Women

In the world of weight-resistance movement, there is a unique difference between women and men. Men tend to wear weight in their upper bodies, and women wear it in their lower bodies. Therefore, men need to be more focused on upper body movements, and women need to be focused on moving their lower bodies.

A basic rule of thumb is this: Men should do two upper body workouts for every lower body workout. Women should do two lower body workouts for every upper body workout.

Action Steps

- ESSENTIAL 1 ACTION: Keep eliminating toxins.
- ESSENTIAL 2 ACTION: Maintain good posture.
- ESSENTIAL 3 ACTION: Keep sticking to the Intermediate Max Diet.
- ESSENTIAL 3 ACTION: Continue all of the other nutrition changes (stay-full, replacement, and multiple-feedings rules, etc.).
- ESSENTIAL 3 ACTION: Keep taking your supplements.
- ESSENTIAL 4 ACTION: Do your SURGE.
- ESSENTIAL 5 ACTION: Plan the war plan; work the war plan.
- ESSENTIAL 5 ACTION: Peace Triathlon, including setting your GPS.

Elite Makeover Challenge

Day 23

Mercury, the Poison (Not the Planet)

Mercury is the second most toxic substance on planet Earth, and for some reason it loves to attach itself to our brains and organs. Therefore, it is important to avoid sources of mercury. Mercury is found in most dental silver-colored (amalgam) fillings. In fact, the fillings are composed of 50 percent mercury. Also, a lot of vaccinations contain mercury. So it's important to discover if you test toxic for mercury or other heavy metals. Your Maximized Living doctor can test you and your family to see how toxic you are.

Remember, you're getting healthier! At this point, you should be working with your medical doctor to be pulling you off or reduce your medications. Do this only with the help of your medical doctor.

Action Steps

Continue all your action steps from the Intermediate Makeover Challenge.

- ESSENTIAL 1 ACTION: Continue to change over any product you put directly on your skin to more organic/natural/toxin-free products.
- ESSENTIAL 1 ACTION: Continue your colon cleanse.
- ESSENTIAL 1 ACTION: Get tested for Mercury toxicity by your Maximized Living Doctor.
- ESSENTIAL 1 AND 3 ACTION: Check your pH balance, eat alkaline foods, and drink greens daily.
- ESSENTIAL 3 ACTION: Keep switching from coffee, soda, and juices to water. Drink your one-half quart of water, using an alkalizing filter for every fifty pounds of body weight, use pH drops and try not to drink anything else.
- ESSENTIAL 3 ACTION: Stick to the Elite Max Diet or eat fewer carbs and replace with more vegetables.
- ESSENTIAL 3 ACTION: Take your recommended supplements.
- ESSENTIAL 4 ACTION: Keep eating a diet in the right proportions.
- ESSENTIAL 4 ACTION: Do your SURGE and/or Pause/Decline weight training.
- ESSENTIAL 5 ACTION: Put on your attitude of gratitude.
- ESSENTIAL 5 ACTION: Meditate during your Peace Triathlon.
- ESSENTIAL 5 ACTION: Sleep in darkness for at least eight hours.

Intermediate Makeover Challenge

Day 24

Inspiration vs. Motivation

As we mentioned way back on day 5, great people are not just motivated short-term by some material gain. Rather than being motivated, those that succeed consistently are inspired. Inspiration is the father of commitment.

Motivation itself is often weak and temporary. It comes only from some short-term desire to win a prize or look or feel differently than you presently do. Again, it is focused on you. Inspiration, however, comes from the burning passion to serve a higher purpose. It is how the drug addict can just say no, the Olympian can go the extra mile, and it is what keeps families and companies happy and together long-term.

Here are some comparisons:

MOTIVATION	INSPIRATION
Driven by personal desires and a need to gain self-satisfaction	Driven by a purpose to make a difference
Can be broken	Can be blocked, but never truly goes away
Ends during tough or inconvenient times	Endures hardship and failure
Yields to excuses	Will not stop until it sees results
Changes with changing emotions	Remains steady. It is stronger than a particular feeling at a particular moment
Is driven by a love for self	Is driven by a love for others
Is like showering or brushing your teeth. You need to do it every day to be successful	Happens once and, while it needs reminders, is there forever

While many succeed through giftedness or luck, the greatest are those that succeed because they were inspired and, thus, committed.

In a particular situation or circumstance where motivation has failed you, describe how inspiration might now make success possible.

_____

_____

Action Steps

- ESSENTIAL 1 ACTION: Stay clean—clean water, clean air, clean food, and clean (drug-free) blood.
- ESSENTIAL 2 ACTION: Keep your power on! Maintain good posture.
- ESSENTIAL 3 ACTION: Remember that continuing the addition rule, multiple feeding rule, stay-full rule, and replacement rule will help you to Meet Fat Sally!
- ESSENTIAL 3 ACTION: Keep sticking to the Intermediate Max Diet.
- ESSENTIAL 3 ACTION: Keep taking your supplements.
- ESSENTIAL 4 ACTION: Do your Pause Sets—chest, biceps, triceps, and abs for a total of ten to twelve minutes of exercise (or move this to a SURGE day). You can count on fifteen to twenty minutes if you add extra exercises for some body parts.
- ESSENTIAL 5 ACTION: Check up from the neck up. Make sure you:

1. Schedule a special time with each family member or your closest friend or relative at least one time a week, and schedule thirty minutes to an hour a day for completely focused time with those closest to you (focused means no television, internet, or answering phones).
2. Schedule daily and weekly time for nutrition (the Big Four) and four to six times a week for exercise.
3. Schedule a daily fifteen-minute Peace Triathlon.

Elite Makeover Challenge

Day 24
Protein

Because healthy proteins are essential for your body's overall health, it's time to start switching over to good proteins. For example, it is time to start switching from grain-fed cows and hormone-filled chickens and turkeys to grass-fed, organic meat, as well as organic dairy, whey and organic, free-range chicken and eggs.

Action Steps

Continue all your action steps from the Intermediate Makeover Challenge.

- ESSENTIAL 1 ACTION: Continue to change over any body product and product you put directly on your skin to more organic/natural/toxin-free products.
- ESSENTIAL 1 ACTION: Continue to switch from toxic cleaning products to natural/organic/healthy products.
- ESSENTIAL 1 ACTION: Continue your colon cleanse.
- ESSENTIAL 1 AND 3 ACTION: Check your pH balance, eat alkaline foods, and drink greens daily.
- ESSENTIAL 3 ACTION: Keep switching from coffee, soda, and juices to water. Drink your one-half quart of water, using an alkalizing filter for every fifty pounds of body weight, use pH drops and try not to drink anything else.
- ESSENTIAL 3 ACTION: Stick to the Elite Max Diet or eat fewer carbs and replace with more vegetables.
- ESSENTIAL 3 ACTION: Keep foods in the right proportions.
- ESSENTIAL 3 ACTION: Take your recommended supplements.
- ESSENTIAL 3 ACTION: Start switching your bad proteins to good proteins.
- ESSENTIAL 4 ACTION: Do your SURGE and/or Pause/Decline/Monster Set weight training.

- ESSENTIAL 5 ACTION: Put on your attitude of gratitude.
- ESSENTIAL 5 ACTION: Meditate during your Peace Triathlon.
- ESSENTIAL 5 ACTION: Sleep in darkness for at least eight hours.

Intermediate Makeover Challenge

Day 25

No Interference

Man cannot make a body. Therefore, man cannot fix a body or truly determine its needs. Right now, no one can tell you what your liver should be doing or how well last night's dinner is digesting. Since we have no idea what is really going on, all we can do is to respect our body, see its vast potential, appreciate its brilliance, and place no interference in its natural path. Your body does not need your help to thrive and survive in this world. How can you help something you could not create or possibly begin to understand? The rule of thumb for Maximized Living is: No interference.

The problem for most of us is figuring out how to stop interfering. Once you place one artificial substance inside of your body or do one thing to disturb its function, simultaneously you get hundreds of thousands of interactions or side effects. However, when left alone, the body always knows precisely what to do to keep or get itself well, without side effects and all of the instructions that come inside of the packaging.

When it comes to the proper operation of your body, everyone knows that stress, lack of exercise, and eating a donut instead of an apple are bad for you. Yet depression, couch potatoes, and candy bars are flourishing anyway. We keep interfering with how we were created to live and function. As a result, many of us now live with or are even born with suffering.

Maximized Living is not simply what you do to look better and lead a better life; it teaches you to stop interfering with the splendid creation called you! If you look back over the past four weeks, you can probably see that the Maximized Living makeover challenges are basically about teaching you how to stop interfering with your body's natural functions or to prevent you from interfering with it in the first place. So keep following the challenges, and stop the interference!

Action Steps

- ESSENTIAL 1 ACTION: Keep eliminating toxins. (Stop interfering!)
- ESSENTIAL 2 ACTION: Maintain good posture.
- ESSENTIAL 3 ACTION: Keep sticking to the Intermediate Max Diet.
- ESSENTIAL 3 ACTION: Continue all of the other nutrition changes (stay-full, replacement, multiple-feedings rules, supplements, etc.).
- ESSENTIAL 4 ACTION: Do your SURGE.

- ESSENTIAL 5 ACTION: Plan the war plan; work the war plan.
- ESSENTIAL 5 ACTION: Continue Peace Triathlon, including setting your GPS.

Elite Makeover Challenge

Day 25
Nutrition/Enzymes

Enzymes are energized protein molecules and play a role in every biochemical reaction in the human body. Life is not possible without enzymes! There are two types of enzymes: digestive enzymes to break food down and metabolic enzymes build the body from what we eat.

Enzymes are sensitive to heat. Even low heat destroys enzymes! Raw vegetables and most fruits are the best way to get enzymes daily, as well as supplementing with enzymes daily.

Action Steps

Continue all your action steps from the Intermediate Makeover Challenge.

- ESSENTIAL 1 ACTION: Continue to change over any body product and product you put directly on your skin to more organic/natural/toxin-free products.
- ESSENTIAL 1 ACTION: Continue to switch from toxic cleaning products to natural/organic/healthy products.
- ESSENTIAL 1 ACTION: Continue your colon cleanse.
- ESSENTIAL 1 AND 3 ACTION: Check your pH balance, eat alkaline foods, and drink greens daily.
- ESSENTIAL 3 ACTION: Keep switching from coffee, soda, and juices to water. Drink your one-half quart of water, using an alkalizing filter for every fifty pounds of body weight, use pH drops and try not to drink anything else.
- ESSENTIAL 3 ACTION: Stick to the Elite Max Diet or eat fewer carbs and replace with more vegetables. Keep foods in the right proportions.
- ESSENTIAL 3 ACTION: Take your recommended supplements.
- ESSENTIAL 3 ACTION: Keep replacing bad proteins with good proteins.
- ESSENTIAL 3 ACTION: Start supplementing with enzymes if your diet does not consist of lots of raw fruits and vegetables.
- ESSENTIAL 4 ACTION: Do your SURGE/weight training.
- ESSENTIAL 5 ACTION: Put on your attitude of gratitude.
- ESSENTIAL 5 ACTION: Meditate during your Peace Triathlon.
- ESSENTIAL 5 ACTION: Sleep in darkness for at least eight hours.

Intermediate Makeover Challenge

Day 26

Overcome Your Addictions: The Ten-Point Reduction Rule

On a scale of one to ten, if a craving is a 10, it will be very hard to resist. On the other hand, if you can get the same craving down to a 7 or 8, you can control that craving some, or most, of the time. If you can get it down even further, you can almost totally control it. If you can reduce a food or beverage craving down below a level 10, such as by drinking decaffeinated tea in the morning instead of coffee, you will have more power over your decisions of what you consume.

For instance, a cup of coffee or two and a donut is a traditional breakfast for many of us. The warmth of coffee and the sweetness of the donut combine to produce a level-10 craving. However, to reduce the higher craving to a much lower one, try substituting herbal tea for the coffee. Select a soothing herbal tea that sounds appetizing, and then add several healthful "extras," such as honey and some rice milk. What will happen to your body's internal feeding system is that it will ingest something similar to coffee. It won't be as good to you as coffee; it won't result in any of that usual "zip" because it contains no caffeine, but it will seem enough like coffee that it will probably tame the coffee craving, if not eliminate it.

You can follow the ten-point reduction rule by figuring out a substitution for any craving and trying it. What have you got to lose, except unwanted toxins, pounds, bad habits, and addictions?

Action Steps

- ESSENTIAL 1 ACTION: Keep eliminating toxins. (Stop interfering!)
- ESSENTIAL 2 ACTION: Maintain good posture.
- ESSENTIAL 3 ACTION: Keep following the Intermediate Max Diet.
- ESSENTIAL 3 ACTION: Keep following the rules—addition, stay-full, multiple-feedings, vacation, and now the ten-point reduction rule.
- ESSENTIAL 3 ACTION: No Sally (Grains, starches such as potatoes, peas, corn, sweet potatoes, flours or sugars) after 3 p.m.
- ESSENTIAL 3 ACTION: Keep taking your supplements.
- ESSENTIAL 4 ACTION: Do your Pause Sets: one exercise each for legs (squat or lunge), calves, shoulders, back/lats for ten to twelve minutes of exercise.
- ESSENTIAL 5 ACTION: Plan the war plan; work the war plan.
- ESSENTIAL 5 ACTION: Continue Peace Triathlon, including setting your GPS

Elite Makeover Challenge

Day 26
Artificial Sweeteners

Artificial sweeteners are chemicals, not food! They have no calories because they don't nourish your body in any way. They are toxins your body has to clear or, depending on how well you detoxify, store. You need to stay clear of these at all costs and start using more natural healthy sweeteners. For example, xylitol, malitol, mannitol, or stevia. These are natural sweeteners that do not trigger an insulin reaction.

Action Steps

Continue all your action steps from the Intermediate Makeover Challenge.

- ESSENTIAL 1 ACTION: Continue to change over any body product and product you put directly on your skin to more organic/natural/toxin-free products.
- ESSENTIAL 1 ACTION: Continue to switch from toxic cleaning products to natural/organic/healthy products.
- ESSENTIAL 1 ACTION: Continue your colon cleanse.
- ESSENTIAL 1 ACTION: Switch your artificial sweeteners to natural sweeteners.
- ESSENTIAL 1 AND 3 ACTION: Check your pH balance, eat alkaline foods, and drink greens daily.
- ESSENTIAL 3 ACTIONS: Keep switching from coffee, soda, and juices to water. Drink your one-half quart of water, using an alkalizing filter for every fifty pounds of body weight, use pH drops and try not to drink anything else.
- ESSENTIAL 3 ACTIONS: Stick to the Elite Max Diet or eat fewer carbs and replace with more vegetables. Keep foods in the right proportions.
- ESSENTIAL 3 ACTIONS: Take your supplements.
- ESSENTIAL 3 ACTIONS: Keep replacing bad proteins with good proteins.
- ESSENTIAL 4 ACTION: Do your SURGE weight training. With surges, you should regularly add an additional round or rounds of SURGE for a total of four or five minutes of actual exercise and still less than twenty minutes total elapsed time.
- ESSENTIAL 5 ACTION: Put on your attitude of gratitude.
- ESSENTIAL 5 ACTION: Meditate during your Peace Triathlon.
- ESSENTIAL 5 ACTION: Sleep in darkness for at least eight hours.

Intermediate Makeover Challenge

Day 27

Sharpen Your Ax

There is no great athlete, composer, business leader, or religious leader who did not have a great teacher. The fastest, least painful way to getting to the top and staying there is to have someone show you the quickest, easiest, most moral way to get there. That's why the next life rule for achieving Maximized Living is so important.

Have Coaches for Everything

Marriage coaches, parenting coaches, financial coaches, sports coaches, and business coaches. Don't make important decisions in your life without consulting the right people. Spend time with your coaches. These are the people to invite over for dinner or ask to go with you on vacations. That way you're not just eating or skiing, you are also becoming a better person. The coaches you surround yourself with sharpen your ax. They make you more capable of moving through life like a well-sharpened ax is able to move better through wood—cleaner, easier, and more effectively.

You don't even have to know some of your coaches personally. They can be authors, lecturers, and business leaders. Go to their seminars, listen to their tapes, and study their organizations as a way of continuing to grow and get sharper until the day you're done getting better.

When is the day that you are done getting better? The day you stop breathing! If you're still breathing, keep getting better.

Action Steps

- ESSENTIAL 1 ACTION: Keep eliminating toxins.
- ESSENTIAL 2 ACTION: Maintain good posture.
- ESSENTIAL 3 ACTION: Keep sticking to the Intermediate Max Diet.
- ESSENTIAL 3 ACTION: Continue all of the other nutrition changes (stay-full, replacement, multiple-feedings, and vacation day rules, etc.).
- ESSENTIAL 3 ACTION: Keep taking your supplements.
- ESSENTIAL 3 ACTION: Follow the ten-point reduction rule to cut back your cravings.
- ESSENTIAL 4 ACTION: Do your SURGE. Look to add an additional surge.

Add another:

Twenty on/twenty recover/twenty on/twenty recover/twenty on for a total of one additional minute of exercise. You can also try going twenty-five to thirty seconds for a SURGE now. IMPORTANT: Do not lose the maximum output. If going over twenty seconds causes you to fade, then stick with twenty.

- ESSENTIAL 5 ACTION: Plan the war plan; work the war plan.
- ESSENTIAL 5 ACTION: Peace Triathlon, including setting your GPS
- ESSENTIAL 5 ACTION: Choose coaches for all of your lives and spend time with them.

Elite Makeover Challenge

Day 27

Antioxidants

Antioxidants are substances or nutrients in our foods that can prevent or slow the oxidative damage to our body. When our body cells use oxygen, they naturally produce free radicals (by-products) that can cause damage. Antioxidants act as "free radical scavengers" and hence prevent and repair damage done by these free radicals. Health problems such as heart disease, diabetes, cancer, and the like are all contributed by oxidative damage. If you're not eating a lot of raw fruits and vegetables, you will need to begin supplementing with antioxidants daily.

Action Steps

Continue all your action steps from the Intermediate Makeover Challenge.

- ESSENTIAL 1 ACTION: Continue to change over any body product and product you put directly on your skin to more organic/natural/toxin-free products.
- ESSENTIAL 1 ACTION: Continue to switch from toxic cleaning products to natural/organic/healthy products.
- ESSENTIAL 1 ACTION: Continue your colon cleanse.
- ESSENTIAL 1 ACTION: Switch your artificial sweeteners to natural sweeteners.
- ESSENTIAL 1 AND 3 ACTION: Check your pH balance, eat alkaline foods, and drink greens daily.
- ESSENTIAL 3 ACTION: Keep switching from coffee, soda, and juices to water. Drink your one-half quart of water, using an alkalizing filter for every fifty pounds of body weight, use pH drops, and try not to drink anything else.
- ESSENTIAL 3 ACTION: Stick to the Elite Max Diet or eat fewer carbs and replace with more vegetables. Keep foods in the right proportions.
- ESSENTIAL 3 ACTION: Take your recommended supplements.
- ESSENTIAL 3 ACTION: Keep replacing bad proteins with good proteins.
- ESSENTIAL 3 ACTION: Start taking an antioxidant supplement daily.
- ESSENTIAL 4 ACTION: Do your SURGE/weight training. Be really looking for progress with total poundage lifted. If the weights have become too light, then you'll stop gaining results.

- ESSENTIAL 5 ACTION: Put on your attitude of gratitude.
- ESSENTIAL 5 ACTION: Meditate during your Peace Triathlon.
- ESSENTIAL 5 ACTION: Sleep in darkness for at least eight hours.

Intermediate Makeover Challenge

Day 28

Don't Smudge Your Lines

A winner without goals and is an eventual loser; a loser with goals is an eventual winner. A great athlete, coach, teacher, carpenter, accountant, painter, doctor, or great anything has goals. No goals = no greatness. Anyone with a future has goals. We have taken a look at goals in several past entries, but now it's time to make a plan to meet you goals.

Here are a few tips:

1. Start by writing down, in detail, all of your dreams and everything you want to accomplish in your time here on this planet.
2. Next, be extremely specific in writing down your strategy for how you are going to achieve each dream (goal). Leave no detail that you can think of unwritten when it comes to what it would take for your dreams to be fulfilled.
3. Once you have completed this list, add these details, your strategy for success, to your weekly war plan. As you follow your plan, commit to doing each of the things exactly as written.
4. Do not smudge your lines. What do we mean by that statement? We mean stick to the plan—exactly. If you said you were going to jog 2 miles, 3 times a week, then jog 2 miles, 3 times per week. If you were going to make 10 sales calls a day, then make at least 10 sales calls per day. Do not skip or shortchange any part of your plan, or you put reaching your goals in jeopardy.

Today, you've already reached one important goal: You have made it through four weeks of the Maximized Living Intermediate Challenge. Put on your favorite tunes, and do a victory dance! We're proud of you, and you should be proud of all you have accomplished on your way to a maximized life. Assess your progress by looking back at day 1. How far have you come?

Action Steps

- ESSENTIAL 1 ACTION: Keep eliminating toxins.
- ESSENTIAL 2 ACTION: Maintain good posture.
- ESSENTIAL 3 ACTION: Keep sticking to the Intermediate Max Diet.

- ESSENTIAL 3 ACTION: Continue all of the other nutrition changes (stay-full, replacement, multiple-feedings, and vacation day rules, etc.).
- ESSENTIAL 3 ACTION: Keep taking your supplements.
- ESSENTIAL 3 ACTION: Follow the ten-point reduction rule to cut back your cravings.
- ESSENTIAL 5 ACTION: Don't smudge your lines. Stick to your goals.
- ESSENTIAL 5 ACTION: Assess your progress over the past four weeks.
- ESSENTIAL 5 ACTION: Plan the war plan; work the war plan.
- ESSENTIAL 5 ACTION: Continue Peace Triathlon, including setting your GPS

Elite Makeover Challenge

Day 28
Changing Your Perception

We create the reality of every interaction we have according to how we perceive what is happening. We may not get to choose what's happening in our life, but we do get to choose how we see what is happening.

The ability to change your perception is one of your greatest human abilities. It means that no matter how difficult your life may become, you will always have the power to rise above and see the positive. It means that you can choose a different perspective on what is happening, one that will enrich your life instead of destroying it.

Action Steps

Continue all your action steps from the Intermediate Makeover Challenge.

- ESSENTIAL 1 ACTION: Continue to change over any body product and product you put directly on your skin to more organic/natural/toxin-free products.
- ESSENTIAL 1 ACTION: Continue to switch from toxic cleaning products to natural/organic/healthy products.
- ESSENTIAL 1 ACTION: Continue your colon cleanse.
- ESSENTIAL 1 ACTION: Keep replacing artificial sweeteners with natural sweeteners.
- ESSENTIAL 1 AND 3 ACTION: Check your pH balance, eat alkaline foods, and drink greens daily.
- ESSENTIAL 3 ACTION: Keep switching from coffee, soda, and juices to water. Drink your one-half quart of water, using an alkalizing filter for every fifty pounds of body weight, use pH drops, and try not to drink anything else.

- ESSENTIAL 3 ACTION: Stick to the Elite Max Diet or eat fewer carbs and replace with more vegetables. Keep foods in the right proportions.
- ESSENTIAL 3 ACTION: Take your recommended supplements.
- ESSENTIAL 3 ACTION: Keep replacing bad proteins with good proteins.
- ESSENTIAL 3 ACTION: Take your antioxidant supplement.
- ESSENTIAL 5 ACTION: Put on your attitude of gratitude.
- ESSENTIAL 5 ACTION: Meditate during your Peace Triathlon.
- ESSENTIAL 5 ACTION: Sleep in darkness for at least eight hours.
- ESSENTIAL 5 ACTION: Write a list of everything that is stressing you out and reverse the way you see it. Find something positive in it, write it down and read it every day.

Intermediate Makeover Challenge

Day 29

Turning Your Goals to Reality

All goals need to be written down and verbalized. There is amazing power in the written and spoken word. Tell other people about your goals so that they can hold you accountable for achieving them. People who are your coaches and mentors are great for helping you to choose, formulate, reformulate, and stick to your plans for reaching your goals and seeing your dreams come true.

Each time you reach a goal, write the word *victory* next to the goal. In addition, have a victory party in honor of your achievement and give yourself a special gift. (Try and make your gifts things like CDs and hiking trips in the mountains rather than pizza and cheesecake. This way you do not end up needing to add the additional goal of losing a hundred pounds by the time you've reached all of your goals!)

By writing out your goals, sharing them with others who can help you reach them, and celebrating your achievements, you can do just about anything!

Action Steps

- ESSENTIAL 1 ACTION: Keep eliminating toxins.
- ESSENTIAL 2 ACTION: Maintain good posture.
- ESSENTIAL 3 ACTION: Keep sticking to the Intermediate Max Diet.
- ESSENTIAL 3 ACTION: Continue all of the other nutrition changes (stay-full, replacement, multiple-feedings, vacation day rules, etc.).
- ESSENTIAL 3 ACTION: Keep taking your supplements.
- ESSENTIAL 3 ACTION: Follow the ten-point reduction rule to cut back your cravings.

- ESSENTIAL 4 ACTION: Do your SURGE for four minutes instead of three.
- ESSENTIAL 5 ACTION: Don't smudge your lines. Stick to your goals.
- ESSENTIAL 5 ACTION: Share your goals with others, and write them down. Celebrate each goal with a victory party or gift to yourself.
- ESSENTIAL 5 ACTION: Plan the war plan; work the war plan.
- ESSENTIAL 5 ACTION: Continue Peace Triathlon, including setting your GPS

Elite Makeover Challenge

Day 29
Going All Out!

This is the Maximized Living Elite Makeover Challenge, so it's time to give it everything you have. It's time to hold yourself to a higher standard than you ever have before. You need to look and evaluate each area of your Maximized Living plan according to the Five Essentials you are now living by and make sure you are going all out to reach your goals.

In order to get what you don't have, you have to do what you've never done!

Action Steps

Continue all your action steps from the Intermediate Makeover Challenge.
Look at every action step below for today and ask yourself, "Am I going all out and doing every step I'm supposed to at the highest level I can?"

- ESSENTIAL 1 ACTION: Continue to change over any body product and product you put directly on your skin to more organic/natural/toxin-free products.
- ESSENTIAL 1 ACTION: Continue to switch from toxic cleaning products to natural/organic/healthy products.
- ESSENTIAL 1 ACTION: Continue your colon cleanse.
- ESSENTIAL 1 ACTION: Keep replacing artificial sweeteners with natural sweeteners.
- ESSENTIAL 1 AND 3 ACTION: Check your pH balance, eat alkaline foods, and drink greens daily.
- ESSENTIAL 3 ACTION: Keep switching from coffee, soda, and juices to water. Drink your one-half quart of water, using an alkalizing filter for every fifty pounds of body weight, use pH drops, and try not to drink anything else.
- ESSENTIAL 3 ACTION: Stick to the Elite Max Diet or eat fewer carbs and replace with more vegetables. Keep foods in the right proportions.

- ESSENTIAL 3 ACTION: Take your recommended supplements.
- ESSENTIAL 3 ACTION: Keep replacing bad proteins with good proteins.
- ESSENTIAL 3 ACTION: Take your antioxidant supplement.
- ESSENTIAL 4 ACTION: Do your SURGE/Pause, Decline, Monster Set weight training.
- ESSENTIAL 5 ACTION: Put on your attitude of gratitude.
- ESSENTIAL 5 ACTION: Meditate during your Peace Triathlon.
- ESSENTIAL 5 ACTION: Sleep in darkness for at least eight hours.
- ESSENTIAL 5 ACTION: Read your positive list.

Intermediate Makeover Challenge

Day 30

Maximized Living for Life

Wow! You did it! When you look back at day 1, can you believe how far you have come in such a short time? The challenge to you from this day forward is to keep going. Your Maximized Living Makeover challenge is not over—far from it. You have only begun a lifelong journey toward health, happiness, and success. As you continue the journey, remember that there is no failure—only times when your focus dims.

We all have times at work, with our relationships, and with our yard and housework when we are not enthusiastic, focused, or doing the things that make these areas successful. However, we do not quit our job, quit on our families, or quit taking care of business – our intensity just dims once in awhile.

Expect to get lost, expect low times, and expect what looks like endings or failures. But by being inspired to live for the people you love and serve and staying the course toward fulfilling your dreams and purpose, you will get back to some degree of commitment and eventually back all the way.

Be inspired for life. We are all counting on you.

Action Steps

- ESSENTIAL 1 ACTION: Keep eliminating toxins. (Stop interfering!)
- ESSENTIAL 2 ACTION: Maintain good posture.
- ESSENTIAL 3 ACTION: Keep following the Intermediate Max Diet.
- ESSENTIAL 3 ACTION: Keep following the rules—addition, stay-full, multiple-feeding, vacation, and the ten-point reduction.
- ESSENTIAL 3 ACTION: No Sally (Grains, starches such as potatoes, peas, corn, sweet potatoes, flours or sugars) after 3:00 p.m.

- ESSENTIAL 3 ACTION: Keep taking your supplements.
- ESSENTIAL 4 ACTION: Do your SURGE for four minutes instead of three.
- ESSENTIAL 5 ACTION: Plan the war plan; work the war plan.
- ESSENTIAL 5 ACTION: Continue Peace Triathlon, including setting your GPS

As you continue to make healthy choices for maximized living, let's stop and evaluate the progress you've made since taking those first body measurements on day 1.

Measure on a scale of 1 to 10 (1 = Terrible, 10 = Excellent)

Overall health

| 1 | 2 | 3 | 4 | 5 | 6 | 7 | 8 | 9 | 10 |

Energy level

| 1 | 2 | 3 | 4 | 5 | 6 | 7 | 8 | 9 | 10 |

Stress level

| 1 | 2 | 3 | 4 | 5 | 6 | 7 | 8 | 9 | 10 |

Attitude (Are you generally happy and positive?)

| 1 | 2 | 3 | 4 | 5 | 6 | 7 | 8 | 9 | 10 |

Time management skills

| 1 | 2 | 3 | 4 | 5 | 6 | 7 | 8 | 9 | 10 |

Spouse/significant other relationship

| 1 | 2 | 3 | 4 | 5 | 6 | 7 | 8 | 9 | 10 |

Relationship with kids

| 1 | 2 | 3 | 4 | 5 | 6 | 7 | 8 | 9 | 10 |

Relationships with others

| 1 | 2 | 3 | 4 | 5 | 6 | 7 | 8 | 9 | 10 |

Financial stability

| 1 | 2 | 3 | 4 | 5 | 6 | 7 | 8 | 9 | 10 |

On course to finding and/or fulfilling your mission in life

| 1 | 2 | 3 | 4 | 5 | 6 | 7 | 8 | 9 | 10 |

Adult Body Mass Index

$$BMI = \left[\frac{WEIGHT\ (pounds)}{Height\ (inches)^2} \right] \times 703$$

WEIGHT IN POUNDS

HEIGHT IN FEET & INCHES	120	130	140	150	160	170	180	190	200	210	220	230	240	250
4'-6"	29	31	34	36	39	41	43	46	48	51	53	56	58	60
4'-8"	27	29	31	34	36	38	40	43	45	47	49	52	54	56
4'-10"	25	27	29	31	34	36	38	40	42	44	46	48	50	52
5'-0"	23	25	27	29	31	33	35	37	39	41	43	45	47	49
5'-2"	22	24	26	27	29	31	33	35	37	38	40	42	44	46
5'-4"	21	22	24	26	28	29	31	33	34	36	38	40	41	43
5'-6"	19	21	23	24	26	27	29	31	32	34	36	37	39	40
5'-8"	18	20	21	23	24	26	27	29	30	32	34	35	37	38
5'-10"	17	19	20	22	23	24	26	27	29	30	32	33	35	36
6'-0"	16	18	19	20	22	23	24	26	27	28	30	31	33	34
6'-2"	15	17	18	19	21	22	23	24	26	27	28	30	31	32
6'-4"	15	16	17	18	20	21	22	23	24	26	27	28	29	30
6'-6"	14	15	16	17	19	20	21	22	23	24	25	27	28	29
6'-8"	13	14	15	17	18	19	20	21	22	23	24	25	26	28

Healthy Weight   Overweight   Obese

			Cholesterol		Body measurements
	Weight		Total		Chest
	Percentage of body fat		HDL		Upper arm
	Blood pressure		LDL		Upper thigh
			Other important blood counts		Waist

Now look at your goals from day 1. How far have you come? If you've come closer, then you're a success. Just keep moving forward one percent at a time, one day at a time. Soon, you'll have a lifetime of Maximized Living!

_____

_____

_____

_____

Elite Makeover Challenge

Day 30

Assess Yourself: Your Overall Update

You did it! You're awesome! You made it to the end of the thirty-day Maximized Living Elite Makeover Challenge, and you are healthier and happier for it, right? Just remember that the journey doesn't stop here. This is just the beginning of a path toward maximized living that you will continue traveling for the rest of your life.

Answer the following questions. Compare your results to where you started on day 1:

_____ BMI

_____ pH

_____ How many days a week did you work out?

_____ How many days did you wake up with gratitude?

_____ How many days did you meditate?

_____ What toxic beverages have you eliminated?

_____ How many cups of water are you drinking per day?

_____ How many days do you go without using microwave?

_____ How many household and personal cleaning products did you switch to natural?

_____ How many days did you take all of your supplements?

Action Steps

- Continue all the action steps from the Intermediate Makeover Challenge.
- Continue all the action steps from the Elite Makeover Challenge.
- Continue your colon cleanse.
- Enjoy your maximized life to the fullest!

PART THREE

If the Maximized Living Makeover challenges have inspired you to make positive changes in your life, we'd love to hear your story. Send us your story at www.MaximizedLivingMakeover.com.

DAY	BREAKFAST	SNACK	LUNCH	SNACK	DINNER	SNACK
		BASIC MEAL PLAN				
1	Whole Grain Cereal (dressed up!)	Celery w/almond butter	Chicken & Veggie Omelet	Cottage cheese& berries	Whole Grain Hamburgers w/ Quinoa Salad	Berries & coconut milk
2	Gluten Free Muffin & fresh fruit	Veggie sticks w/ Ranch	Egg Salad on Ezekiel Bread	Pita Chips & Hummus	Coconut Chicken Tenders w/peas	Spelt Cookies
3	Gluten Free Pancakes w/Strawberries	Caprice Salad	Chicken Salad on Greens	Mixed Nuts	Lamb Chops w/ Roast vegetables	Fresh Fruit Salad
4	Whole Grain Bagel w/Almond Butter	Melons	Beef - Vegetable Soup	Celery w/Almond Butter	Stir-fry Vegetables w/ Chicken	Raw Cheese & Nuts
5	Eggs Florentine w/ Turkey Bacon	Whole Grain Pretzels	Stuffed Peppers	Cottage cheese & berries	Pot Roast w/Green Salad	Homemade Ice Cream
6	Breakfast Burrito (in whole grain wrap)	Gluten Free Muffin	Vegetarian Chili	Caprice Salad	Meat Loaf w/Sweet potato	Raw Cheese & WG Crackers
7	Cheesy -Curry Eggs w/ Beef Sausage	Mixed Nuts	Eggplant - Tomato Bake	Veggie sticks w/ Ranch	Leftovers!	Melons
8	Greens & Berry Shake	Raw Cheese& WG Crackers	Whole Grain Vegetable Wrap	Fresh Fruit	Italian Tilapia w/ Caprice Salad	Celery w/Almond Butter
9	Whole Grain Cereal (dressed up!)	Mellons	Egg Salad on Ezekiel Bread	Cottage cheese & berries	Coconut Chicken Tenders w/peas	Raw Cheese & WG Crackers
10	Gluten Free Pancakes w/Strawberries	Veggie sticks w/ Ranch	Chicken Salad on Greens	Pita Chips & Hummus	Lamb Chops w/ Roast vegetables	Fresh Fruit Salad
11	Eggs Florentine w/ Turkey Bacon	Caprice Salad	Vegetarian Chili	Mixed Nuts	Stir-fry Vegetables w/ Chicken	Homemade Ice Cream
12	Breakfast Burrito (in whole grain wrap)	Whole Grain Pretzels	Eggplant - Tomato Bake	Celery w/Almond Butter	Meat Loaf w/Sweet potato	Spelt Cookies

BASIC MEAL PLAN

DAY	BREAKFAST	SNACK	LUNCH	SNACK	DINNER	SNACK
13	Gluten Free Muffin & fresh fruit	Celery w/Almond Butter	Beef - Vegetable Soup	Cottage cheese & berries	Leftovers!	Herbal tea
14	Whole Grain Cereal (dressed up!)	Raw Cheese& WG Crackers	Chicken Salad on Greens	Fresh Fruit	Pot Roast w/Green Salad	Celery w/Almond Butter
15	Greens & Berry Shake	Veggie sticks w/ Ranch	Egg Salad on Ezekiel Bread	Pita Chips & Hummus	Italian Tilapia w/ Caprice Salad	Berries & coconut milk
16	Cheesy -Curry Eggs w/ Beef Sausage	Melons	Stuffed Peppers	Mixed Nuts	Lamb Chops w/ Roast vegetables	Raw Cheese & WG Crackers
17	Eggs Florentine w/ Turkey Bacon	Gluten Free muffin	Eggplant - Tomato Bake	Veggie sticks w/ Ranch	Coconut Chicken Tenders w/peas	Fresh Fruit Salad
18	Gluten Free Muffin & fresh fruit	Caprice Salad	Whole Grain Vegetable Wrap	Pita Chips & Hummus	Meat Loaf w/Sweet potato	Melons
19	Breakfast Burrito (in whole grain wrap)	Mixed Nuts	Chicken Salad on Greens	Cottage cheese & berries	Leftovers!	Herbal tea
20	Whole Grain Cereal (dressed up!)	Melons	Vegetarian Chili	Celery w/Almond Butter	Pot Roast w/Green Salad	Spelt Cookies
21	Gluten Free Pancakes w/Strawberries	Celery w/Almond Butter	Beef - Vegetable Soup	Fresh Fruit	Italian Tilapia w/ Caprice Salad	Raw Cheese & WG Crackers
22	Cheesy -Curry Eggs w/ Beef Sausage	Whole Grain Pretzels	Eggplant - Tomato Bake	Pita Chips & Hummus	Stir-fry Vegetables w/ Chicken	Berries & coconut milk
23	Greens & Berry Shake	Veggie sticks w/ Ranch	Egg Salad on Ezekiel Bread	Mixed Nuts	Coconut Chicken Tenders w/peas	Homemade Ice Cream
24	Eggs Florentine w/ Turkey Bacon	Raw Cheese& WG Crackers	Stuffed Peppers	Veggie sticks w/ Ranch	Lamb Chops w/ Roast vegetables	Melons
25	Breakfast Burrito (in whole grain wrap)	Caprice Salad	Whole Grain Vegetable Wrap	Pita Chips & Hummus	Leftovers!	Fresh Fruit Salad
26	Whole Grain Cereal (dressed up!)	Gluten Free muffin	Chicken Salad on Greens	Celery w/Almond Butter	Pot Roast w/Green Salad	Spelt Cookies
27	Gluten Free Pancakes w/Strawberries	Celery w/Almond Butter	Vegetarian Chili	Cottage cheese & berries	Italian Tilapia w/ Caprice Salad	Herbal tea
28	Gluten Free Muffin & fresh fruit	Veggie sticks w/ Ranch	Beef - Vegetable Soup	Pita Chips & Hummus	Meat Loaf w/Sweet potato	Homemade Ice Cream
29	Greens & Berry Shake	Melons	Egg Salad on Ezekiel Bread	Caprice Salad	Stir-fry Vegetables w/ Chicken	Berries & coconut milk
30	Eggs Florentine w/ Turkey Bacon	Caprice Salad	Stuffed Peppers	Celery w/Almond Butter	Leftovers!	Melons
31	Cheesy -Curry Eggs w/ Beef Sausage	Gluten Free muffin	Eggplant - Tomato Bake	Mixed Nuts	Coconut Chicken Tenders w/peas	Herbal tea
32	Gluten Free Pancakes w/Strawberries	Raw Cheese& WG Crackers	Beef - Vegetable Soup	Fresh Fruit	Italian Tilapia w/ Caprice Salad	Raw Cheese & WG Crackers
33	Greens & Berry Shake	Celery w/Almond Butter	Chicken Salad on Greens	Veggie sticks w/ Ranch	Meat Loaf w/Sweet potato	Spelt Cookies
34	Whole Grain Cereal (dressed up!)	Melons	Egg Salad on Ezekiel Bread	Pita Chips & Hummus	Lamb Chops w/ Roast vegetables	Herbal tea
35	Gluten Free Muffin & fresh fruit	Veggie sticks w/ Ranch	Vegetarian Chili	Cottage cheese & berries	Pot Roast w/Green Salad	Fresh Fruit Salad

ADVANCED MEAL PLAN

DAY	BREAKFAST	SNACK	LUNCH	SNACK	DINNER	SNACK
1	Eggs Florentine & Turkey Bacon	Apple Crisp	Taco-Mex Salad	Red Cabbage & Guacamole	Stir-Fry Vegetables w/ Chicken	Raw Cheese & Nuts
2	Breakfast Burrito (in Hemp Wrap)	Grapefruit	Beef-Veg Soup	Raw Cheese & Nuts	Coconut Chicken Tenders w/Peas	1/2 Avocado w/Salt & Lime
3	Cheesy-Curry Eggs & Beef Sausage	Lemon Parfait	Broccoli Burgers	Veggie Sticks & Ranch	Stuffed Peppers II	Nuts, Seeds & Coconut Flakes
4	Greens & Berry Shake	Raw Cheese & Nuts	Veggie Omelet	Berry Shake	Italian Tilapia w/ Green Salad	Red Cabbage & Guacamole
5	Salad! (greens are always good!)	Cottage Cheese & Berries	Eggplant-Tomato Bake	1/2 Avocado w/Salt & Lime	Meat Loaf w/Roast Vegetables	Veggie Sticks & Ranch
6	Yogurt & Fresh Berries w/Coconut	Red Pepper & Hummus	Leftovers!	Nuts, Seeds & Coconut Flakes	Curried Lamb on Roast Eggplant	Lemon Parfait
7	Breakfast Burrito (in Hemp Wrap)	Grapefruit	Broccoli Burgers	1/2 Avocado w/Salt & Lime	Coconut Chicken Tenders w/Peas	Veggie Sticks & Ranch
8	Cheesy-Curry Eggs & Beef Sausage	Apple Crisp	Eggplant-Tomato Bake	Veggie Sticks & Ranch	Leftovers!	Red Cabbage & Guacamole
9	Yogurt & Fresh Berries w/Coconut	Raw Cheese & Nuts	Beef-Veg Soup	Berry Shake	Stuffed Peppers II	Nuts, Seeds & Coconut Flakes
10	Eggs Florentine & Turkey Bacon	Lemon Parfait	Taco-Mex Salad	Red Cabbage & Guacamole	Stir-Fry Vegetables w/ Chicken	Veggie Sticks & Ranch
11	Salad! (greens are always good!)	Grapefruit	Leftovers!	Raw Cheese & Nuts	Italian Tilapia w/ Green Salad	Lemon Parfait
12	Breakfast Burrito (in Hemp Wrap)	Cottage Cheese & Berries	Veggie Omelet	Nuts, Seeds & Coconut Flakes	Coconut Chicken Tenders w/Peas	Red Cabbage & Guacamole
13	Cheesy-Curry Eggs & Beef Sausage	Apple Crisp	Beef-Veg Soup	1/2 Avocado w/Salt & Lime	Leftovers!	Veggie Sticks & Ranch
14	Greens & Berry Shake	Raw Cheese & Nuts	Broccoli Burgers	Veggie Sticks & Ranch	Stuffed Peppers II	Lemon Parfait
15	Yogurt & Fresh Berries w/Coconut	Red Pepper & Hummus	Eggplant-Tomato Bake	Red Cabbage & Guacamole	Curried Lamb on Roast Eggplant	Raw Cheese & Nuts
16	Eggs Florentine & Turkey Bacon	Grapefruit	Taco-Mex Salad	Berry Shake	Coconut Chicken Tenders w/Peas	Nuts, Seeds & Coconut Flakes
17	Salad! (greens are always good!)	Lemon Parfait	Veggie Omelet	Raw Cheese & Nuts	Meat Loaf w/Roast Vegetables	1/2 Avocado w/Salt & Lime
18	Breakfast Burrito (in Hemp Wrap)	Apple Crisp	Leftovers!	Nuts, Seeds & Coconut Flakes	Stir-Fry Vegetables w/ Chicken	Red Cabbage & Guacamole
19	Cheesy-Curry Eggs & Beef Sausage	Cottage Cheese & Berries	Taco-Mex Salad	Raw Cheese & Nuts	Italian Tilapia w/ Green Salad	Lemon Parfait
20	Eggs Florentine & Turkey Bacon	Lemon Parfait	Broccoli Burgers	Red Cabbage & Guacamole	Leftovers!	Veggie Sticks & Ranch
21	Yogurt & Fresh Berries w/Coconut	Raw Cheese & Nuts	Eggplant-Tomato Bake	Veggie Sticks & Ranch	Stuffed Peppers II	Lemon Parfait
22	Greens & Berry Shake	Red Pepper & Hummus	Veggie Omelet	1/2 Avocado w/Salt & Lime	Coconut Chicken Tenders w/Peas	Raw Cheese & Nuts
23	Breakfast Burrito (in Hemp Wrap)	Grapefruit	Leftovers!	Nuts, Seeds & Coconut Flakes	Meat Loaf w/Roast Vegetables	1/2 Avocado w/Salt & Lime

ADVANCED MEAL PLAN

DAY	BREAKFAST	SNACK	LUNCH	SNACK	DINNER	SNACK
24	Yogurt & Fresh Berries w/Coconut	Red Pepper & Hummus	Broccoli Burgers	Raw Cheese & Nuts	Stir-Fry Vegetables w/ Chicken	Red Cabbage & Guacamole
25	Cheesy-Curry Eggs & Beef Sausage	Lemon Parfait	Taco-Mex Salad	Red Cabbage & Guacamole	Leftovers!	Veggie Sticks & Ranch
26	Salad! (greens are always good!)	Apple Crisp	Eggplant-Tomato Bake	1/2 Avocado w/Salt & Lime	Stuffed Peppers II	Raw Cheese & Nuts
27	Eggs Florentine & Turkey Bacon	Cottage Cheese & Berries	Beef-Veg Soup	Berry Shake	Italian Tilapia w/ Green Salad	Red Cabbage & Guacamole
28	Yogurt & Fresh Berries w/Coconut	Raw Cheese & Nuts	Veggie Omelet	1/2 Avocado w/Salt & Lime	Meat Loaf w/Roast Vegetables	Lemon Parfait
29	Greens & Berry Shake	Red Pepper & Hummus	Leftovers!	Veggie Sticks & Ranch	Coconut Chicken Tenders w/Peas	Raw Cheese & Nuts
30	Breakfast Burrito (in Hemp Wrap)	Lemon Parfait	Broccoli Burgers	Berry Shake	Curried Lamb on Roast Eggplant	Red Cabbage & Guacamole
31	Yogurt & Fresh Berries w/Coconut	Grapefruit	Taco-Mex Salad	Red Cabbage & Guacamole	Stuffed Peppers II	Veggie Sticks & Ranch
32	Salad! (greens are always good!)	Cottage Cheese & Berries	Beef-Veg Soup	Nuts, Seeds & Coconut Flakes	Stir-Fry Vegetables w/ Chicken	1/2 Avocado w/Salt & Lime
33	Eggs Florentine & Turkey Bacon	Apple Crisp	Leftovers!	Raw Cheese & Nuts	Meat Loaf w/Roast Vegetables	Red Cabbage & Guacamole
34	Greens & Berry Shake	Raw Cheese & Nuts	Broccoli Burgers	Veggie Sticks & Ranch	Italian Tilapia w/ Green Salad	Lemon Parfait
35	Cheesy-Curry Eggs & Beef Sausage	Lemon Parfait	Eggplant-Tomato Bake	Berry Shake	Coconut Chicken Tenders w/Peas	Raw Cheese & Nuts

Notes

1. "American Healthcare Is Among the Worst in the Industrialized World. How Can We Do Better?," *Discover*, May 2007, 68.

2. Commonwealth Study, http://www.cmwf.org (accessed February 20, 2008).

3. "What Scares Doctors Most? Being the Patient!," *Time*, May 1, 2006, 43.

4. Carey, John, "Medical Guesswork," BusinessWeek Online, May 29, 2008.

5. California Department of Developmental Services, "2003 DDS Autism Report," http://www.dds.ca.gov/autism (accessed February 20, 2008).

6. Centers for Disease Control, Autism and Developmental Disabilities Monitoring Network, "Morbidity and Mortality Weekly Report: Prevalence of Autism Spectrum Disorders," February 9, 2007, http://www.cdc.gov/MMWR/preview/mmwrhtml/ss5601a2.htm (accessed February 20, 2008).

7. Centers for Disease Control, "New Data on Autism Spectrum Disorders," February 9, 2007, http://www.cdc.gov/od/oc/media/pressrel/2007/r070208.htm (accessed February 20, 2008).

8. Langreth, Robert, "Just Say No," *Forbes*, November 29, 2004.

9. O. LAVIE, *et al*, "The Risk of Developing Uterine Sarcoma After Tamoxifen Use," International Journal of Gynecological Cancer OnlineEarly Articles, doi:10.1111/j.1525-1438.2007.01025.x.

10. Centers for Disease Control, "Vaccine Excipient and Media Summary," http://www.cdc.gov/vaccines/pubs/pinkbook/downloads/appendices/B/excipient-table-1.pdf, http://www.cdc.gov/vaccines/pubs/pinkbook/downloads/appendices/B/excipient-table-2.pdf (accessed December 6, 2007) A. S. Khan, "FDA Vaccines and Related Biological Products Advisory Committee: Adventitious Agent Testing of Novel Cell Substrates for Vaccine Manufacture," U. S. Food and Drug Administration, November 16, 2005, http://www.fda.gov/ohrms/dockets/ac/05/slides/5-4188S1_3.ppt (accessed February 20, 2008); Johns Hopkins School of Public Health, Institute for Vaccine Safety, www.VaccineSafety.edu, "Excipients and Allergens in Vaccines," http://www.vaccinesafety.edu/components-Excipients.htm (accessed December 6, 2007); and http://www.vaccinesafety.edu/components-Allergens.htm (accessed December 6, 2007).

11. U.S. Environmental Protection Agency, "Mercury Laws and Regulations," www.EPA.gov, http://www.epa.gov/epaoswer/hazwaste/mercury/regs.htmNo. hazwaste (accessed December 6, 2007); and National Vaccine Information Center, "The Mercury Calculator," http://www.nvic.org./Issues/HgCalculator (accessed December 6, 2007).

12. G. L. Klein, A. C. Alfrey, *et al*, "Working Group on Standards for Aluminum Content of Parenteral Nutrition Solutions," *American Journal of Clinical Nutrition*, Journal of Parenteral and Enteral Nutrition, Vol 15, Issue 2, 194-198, March 15, 1991 by American Society for Parenteral and Enteral Nutrition, http://jpen.aspenjournals.org/cgi/content/abstract/15/2/194 (accessed December 6, 2007).

13. American Academy of Pediatrics. *Pediatrics*: Report of the Committee on the Control of Infectious Diseases (Red Book – 19th Edition). 1982. https://owa016.msoutlookonline.net/owa/?ae=Item&a=New&t=IPM.Note#_ednref1 (accessed February 29, 2008)

14. Centers for Disease Control, "Morbidity and Mortality Weekly Report: Recommended Immunization Schedules for Persons Aged 0–18 Years—United States, 2007," January 5, 2007, http://www.cdc.gov/mmwr/preview/mmwrhtml/mm5551a7.htm?s_cid=mm5551a7_e (accessed February 20, 2008).

15. Daily News Archive, "CDC Report Reveals Americans' Exposure to Environmental Chemicals," February 4, 2003, http://www.beyondpesticides.org/news/daily_news_archive/2003/2_4_03.htm (accessed February 20, 2008)

16. American Journal of Pain Management, AJPM 1994; 4:36-39

17. S. Haldeman, "Neurologic Effects of the Adjustment," *Journal of Manipulative and Physiological Therapeutics*, February, 2000, Volume 23, Number 2, page 3; C. A. Lantz, "The Vertebral Subluxation Complex (Part 2): The Neurophysiological and Myopathological Components," *Chiropractic Research Journal*, 1990, 1 (4); P. Bolton, "Reflex Effects of Vertebral Subluxations: The Peripheral Nervous System," *Journal of Manipulative and Physiological Therapeutics*, 2000 23 (2); The Association of Chiropractic Colleges Guidelines for Subluxation: A subluxation is a complex of functional and/or structural and/or pathological articular changes that compromise neural integrity and may influence organ system function and general health, *Journal of Vertebral Subluxation Research*, March 6, 2006.

18. J. D. Grostic, "Dentate Ligament-Cord Distortion Hypothesis," *Chiropractic Research Journal* 1988 1(1): 47–55; H. S. Crow and T. Kleinman, "Upper Cervical Influence on the Reticular System," *The Upper Cervical Monograph*, 1991 5(1): 12–14; K. Abbot, "Foramen Magnum and High Cervical Cord Lestions Simulating Degenerative Disease of the Nervous System," *Ohio State Medical Journal*, July, 1950 46: 645–647; R. Sweat and T. Sievert, "Chiropractic and Vertebral Arteries (Parts 1 and 2)," *Today's Chiropractic*, September/October 1984, 45–48; November/December 1984, 23–24.

19. A. Lantz, "The Subluxation Complex in: Foundations of Chiropractic: Subluxation," Meridel Gatterman, Ed. *Mosby Year Book*. January 1995; C. A. Lantz, "Immobilization Degeneration and the Fixation Hypothesis of the Chiropractic Subluxation," *Chiropractic Research Journal* vol. 1, no. 1., 1988.

[20] Deborah M. Kado, MD, Arun S. Karlamangla, MD, Elizabeth Barrett-Connor, MD and Gail A. Greendale, MD, Hyperkyphotic Posture Predicts Mortality in Older Community-Dwelling Men and Women: A Prospective Study," *Journal of the American Geriatrics Society*, Vol. 52 Issue 10 Pp. 1662- October 2004. 21. Shimizu, Kentaro MD, "Spinal Kyphosis Causes Demyelination and Neuronal Loss in the Spinal Cord," *Spine* vol. 30(21), November 1, 2005, 2388–2392.

[22] L. E. Koch, "Tissue distribution of components of the insulin-like growth factor system in sudden infant death and controls," *Forensic Science Int*, October 12, 1998:97 (1):1–9; L. E. Koch *et al*, *Liliencronweg* 6, D-24340, Eckernforde, Germany; Gilles, *American Journal Disabled Child*, 133:30, 979; Schneier, M, Burns, Atlanto-Occipital Hypermobility in Sudden Infant Death Syndrome," *Journal of Chiropractic Research and Clinical Investigation*, Vol. 7, No. 2, July 1, 1991.

[23] I. A., Kapandji, The Physiology of the Joints, Volume 1, May 31, 2007, Churchill Livingstone, 6th Edition.

[24] This study, published in the *Journal of Vertebral Subluxation Research*, was reported in *Medical News Today*, http://www.medicalnewstoday.com/medicalnews.php?newsid=20809 (accessed February 20, 2008).

[25] Thiel, Haymo W. DC, PhD; Bolton, Jennifer E. PhD; Docherty, Sharon PhD; Portlock, Jane C. PhD, "Safety of Chiropractic Manipulation of the Cervical Spine: A Prospective National Survey," *Spine Medical Journal*, October 1, 2007, 32(21):2375–2378.

[26] Committee on Identifying and Preventing Medication Errors, Philip Aspden, et al, July 20, 2006, National Academies, *Preventing Medication Errors: Quality Chasm Series*, The National Academies Press, Washington DC, 2007.

[27] To see specific spinal hygiene programs, go to "Straighten Up, America"; Copyright © 2003 Life University, College of Chiropractic, College of Arts and Sciences; http://www.life.edu/spinalhygiene/index.html; http://www.life.edu/Press_Room/Straighten_Up_America_Becomes_the_National_Spinal_Health_Promotion_Program.pdf "Straighten Up America Becomes the National PublicEducation Program for Spinal Health on World Spine Day," October 6, 2006 (accessed February 20, 2008).

[28] C. Shepeher, BS, DC and Ron Kirk, BS, Ed., MA, DC, "Spinal Hygiene and its Impact on Health and General Well-being," *Journal of Vertebral Subluxation Research*, August 16, 2004.

[29] Committee on Identifying and Preventing Medication Errors, Philip Aspden, et al, July 20, 2006, National Academies, *Preventing Medication Errors: Quality Chasm Series*, The National Academies Press, Washington DC, 2007.

[30] "Why Grassfed Animal Products are Better For You," http://www.texasgrassfedbeef.com/omega_3_fatty_acids.htm (accessed February 29, 2008)

[31] Patricia Kane, PhD, "It's All In the Fat," October 8, 2003, http://prohealthnetwork.com/library/showarticle.cfm/id/1675/searchtext/efas/ (accessed February 20, 2008).

[32] Knopp, Robert H. and Retzlaff, Barbara M., "Saturated fat prevents coronary artery disease? An American paradox," American Journal of Clinical Nutrition, Vol. 80, No. 5, 1102-1103, November 2004.

[33] Bender, R., C. Trautnet, M. Spraul, and M. Berger. 1998. Assessment of excess mortality in obesity. Am. J. Epidemiol. 147 (1): 42-48

[34] Stuart, Julia, "What Makes Us Fat?" The London Independent, August 28, 2007; Among the findings presented by researchers at Columbia University in New York at the annual meeting of the North American Association for the Study of Obesity, in partnership with the American Diabetes Association; http://findarticles.com/p/articles/mi_qn4158/is_20070828/ai_n20523393/print (accessed February 29, 2008)

[35] British Journal of Sports Medicine April 2001;35:114-117

[36] Steven Blair, P.E.D., "Fitness, not Fatness, is the Issue," WELL Newsletter for Wellness, Volume 1, Issue II, Fall, 1999.

[37] Environmental Protection Agency EPA, Office Radiation and Indoor Air, Indoor Environment Division, http://epa.gov/air/basic.html and http://www.natlallergy.com/article.asp?ai=133 (accessed February 29, 2008)

About the Authors

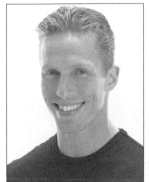

Dr. Ben Lerner

is America's Maximized-Living Mentor. He is the author of the New York Times, Wall Street Journal, and Christian Booksellers Association best-selling book, *Body by God: the Owner's Manual for Maximized Living*. His breakthrough strategies for total health and well-being are the foundation to his thriving local practice, which is a center for maximized living, and one of the largest clinics of any kind in the world. An academic all-American wrestler in college, he has served as physician for the US wrestling teams in six World Team competitions and two Olympiads. At seminars, conferences, and media appearances throughout North America, he shows people how to apply the four laws of Olympic success to achieve optimal health, outrageous happiness, and prosperity. Dr. Lerner lives in Celebration, Florida with his wife, Dr. Sheri Lerner. He is the proud father of Skylar, Nicole, and Cael.

www.MaximizedLivingDrBLerner.com

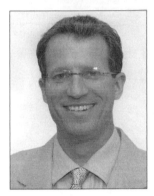

Co-author Greg Loman

Dr. Greg Loman is the co-author of *the New York Times* Best-Selling book, *One Minute* Wellness. A radio and television personality through his Ultimate Health broadcasts in Naples, Florida. He is a health and performance expert, speaking to churches and businesses around the U.S. as well as consulting for their leaders. An off-shore world power boat racing champion, Dr. Greg has learned what it takes to be the very best. He cofounded Teach the World about Chiropractic with Dr. Ben Lerner. Their clients have the largest, most successful clinics in the profession today. He is married to Dr. Maryella Loman and has two children, Ki and Jadyn.

www.MaximizedLivingDrLoman.com

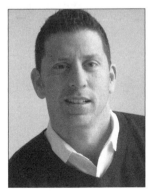

Co-author Charles Majors

Dr. Charles Majors has built five health-care clinics, one of which is among the largest natural health-care clinics in the world. He consults and coaches doctors, patients, and businesses on how to apply the principles of Maximized Living to achieve outrageous health and incredible happiness. He is married to Andrea and has three children, Caleb, Austin, and Reese.

www.MaximizedLivingDrMajors.com

Proven tools to create real "healthy longevity"

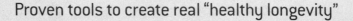

FREE BONUS

Two tickets to the Maximized Living Makeover seminar.

[a $297 value]

Nutrition, fitness, stress management, time management, and the 4 rules of olympic success to:

- customized diets based on your hormones
- lower cholesterol without dangerous medications
- toxicity testing and how to eliminate toxic effects on your weight
- test your body fat and metabolism
- get in the shape of your life with only 12 minutes of exercise — per week!
- time management — get 160 hours out of a 40-hour week
- say goodbye to stress, worry, and fear
- more than double your energy

To collect your free tickets, **visit www.maximizedlivingmakeover.com**
[click on "free tickets"]